Rehabilitation Resource Manual

VISION

Resources for Rehabilitation
Lexington, Massachusetts

This book is part of the

"Living with Low Vision Series"

Other publications in the series include:

Living with Low Vision
A Resource Guide for People with Sight Loss
(LARGE PRINT)

Providing Services for People with Vision Loss
A Multidisciplinary Perspective
Susan L. Greenblatt, Editor
(Standard print and cassette)

Meeting the Needs of People with Vision Loss
A Multidisciplinary Perspective
Susan L. Greenblatt, Editor
(Standard print and cassette)

Resources for Rehabilitation
33 Bedford Street, Suite 19A
Lexington, MA 02173

Rehabilitation Resource Manual: VISION, fourth edition

ISBN 0-929718-10-0

TABLE OF CONTENTS

INTRODUCTION

The simultaneous increase in the population with visual impairments and rapid advances in technology have served as the impetus for producing a wide variety of products and services that enable people with visual impairments to function independently. Despite the technological advances, many individuals with visual impairments never learn about these services and products. Health care professionals and other service providers often are not educated about the availability of these services and devices; therefore, they are unable to refer their patients or clients for much needed help.

This book was written for the many health care professionals, rehabilitation professionals, psychologists, social workers, educators, information and referral specialists, and librarians who provide a vast array of services to individuals with vision loss. It is intended to help these professionals make specific referrals that are appropriate for the needs of the people they serve.

Although providing referrals for individuals with visual impairments is a major goal of this volume, another broader goal is to provide information that enables professionals in the various fields that serve people with vision loss to learn how to work together to ensure that their clients/patients/students receive coordinated services. The case vignettes that have been added to this edition of the Manual are intended to illustrate multidisciplinary cooperation in providing services to individuals who are visually impaired or blind.

The Manual includes introductory narrative material on each topic as well as annotated listings. Professional organizations include membership organizations and organizations that provide services to professionals. Research organizations include organizations that either fund or conduct research related to eye disease, the effects of vision loss, the development of assistive devices, or rehabilitation. Professional publications include books and articles intended for a professional audience. In order to guarantee that information provided in directories is up-to-date, only those directories that had current information at the time of publication of this book or those that are updated regularly are included.

Following the professional listings are Referral Resources. These listings describe organizations, publications and tapes, and assistive devices that are useful to people with vision loss. Publications that are generally available in book stores or libraries include the publisher's name only. Other publications include a mailing address as well. Listings of organizations and publications are alphabetical within sections. All of the material is up to date and prices were accurate as of the time of publication. However, it is always a good idea to check with publishers and manufacturers to ascertain the availability and current price of their publications and products. All prices listed are in U.S. funds, unless otherwise noted.

The phone numbers of organizations that have special telephone access for people with hearing impairments or speech impairments, formerly called telecommunications devices for the deaf, are now called text telephones and are followed by (TT) in the listings. When the same number is available for either voice or TT access, (V/TT) appears after the phone number. FAX numbers are also included when available.

The <u>Manual</u> is updated on a regular basis. Send suggestions of additional information that should be included in the <u>Manual</u> to:

Editor, Rehabilitation Resource Manual: VISION
Resources for Rehabilitation
33 Bedford Street, Suite 19A
Lexington, MA 02173

Chapter 1

VISION LOSS: AN OVERVIEW

THE EXPANDING POPULATION

Professionals who work with people with vision loss and those who study this topic often lament the lack of accurate statistics on the prevalence of visual impairment. The number of people with visual impairments; the severity of the visual impairments they experience; and the etiology and type of impairments have not been estimated with the degree of accuracy necessary for policy-makers or service providers. Yet virtually all in the field would agree that the population with visual impairments has increased dramatically in recent years.

Two major factors have contributed to the increase in visual impairment. First, advances in technology have enabled very low birth weight babies to survive, often with serious disabilities including visual impairment. Second, the number of older people, who account for a large portion of the population with vision loss, has increased rapidly. It is projected that the older population will continue to grow and that by the year 2030, there will be 65.6 million Americans 65 years or older (Fowles: 1991).

Data from the U.S. Census Bureau (1986) indicate that nearly 13 million Americans age 15 years or older report having problems reading ordinary newsprint, even with the use of corrective lenses. Because this statistic represents a self-report of visual impairment, it does not provide a standardized measure; nonetheless, it does suggest that visual impairment is one of the major physical disabilities in the U.S. Of ten impairments studied by the U.S. National Center for Health Statistics (1981), visual impairment had the second highest prevalence rate and the largest rate of increase from 1971 to 1977.

A recent study of individuals age 40 or over living in East Baltimore suggests that less than normal visual acuity is often attributable to improper refraction. Proper refraction improved visual acuity by at least one line on the Snellen acuity chart in 54% of the population and by three or more lines for 7.5% of the population (Tielsch et al.: 1991). The same study also found that blacks were less likely than whites to have had surgery for glaucoma. Blacks were also less likely than whites to have had surgery for senile cataracts. These findings indicate that blacks were more likely than whites to experience blindness that could have been prevented (Sommer et al.: 1991).

In Canada, there are 552,580 citizens age 15 and over who are unable to read ordinary newsprint or to see someone from four meters, even when wearing glasses (Statistics Canada: 1988). This figure represents 18% of the total disabled population age 15 and older. Sixty percent of Canadians who are visually impaired or blind and registered with the Canadian National Institute for the Blind are age 65 or older (CNIB: 1985).

The increase in the population with visual impairments is reflected in the number of visits to ophthalmologists' offices. Recent data indicate that visits to ophthalmologists increased by 30% from 1980 to 1985 and that this increase is largely attributable to the aging of the population (NCHS: 1989). The same survey found that visits for retinal problems (mainly macular degeneration) and cataracts more than doubled during this period and that visits for glaucoma also increased dramatically. A study of ambulatory care found that there were nearly 44 million visits to ophthalmologists in 1990, representing the highest number of visits to a nonprimary care specialist; nearly one in five Americans (17.8%) visited an ophthalmologist during the year (Schappert: 1992). Another recent survey of practicing ophthalmologists (Greenblatt: 1988a) found that, on average, ophthalmologists see 21 patients per week with visual impairments, defined as corrected acuity of less than 20/20 in the better eye to no useful vision.

UNDERSTANDING THE RESPONSES TO VISION LOSS

When individuals experience vision loss, they experience a wide range of emotional responses including shock, denial, fear, anger, and depression. All of these responses are normal. Ultimately, most individuals accept their vision loss and make adjustments that allow for an independent lifestyle.

An individual's responses to vision loss will be shaped by a lifetime's experience of responses to other difficult or stressful situations. Those individuals who have coped well with other situations can be expected to face vision loss in the same manner. The severity of the impairment and whether it occurred gradually or suddenly may also affect the individual's responses.

Vision loss affects all aspects of life. Individuals who have experienced vision loss fear that they will lose their jobs and their ability to support themselves; that they will be unable to take care of themselves; and that they will become the object of pity. Vision loss threatens the individual's independence, which in turn diminishes self-esteem. When self-esteem is low, it is often difficult to accept assistance offered by others, including services from professionals.

Individuals with vision loss often need time to adjust psychologically before they are able to begin the rehabilitation process. The amount of time that individuals need before they accept their vision loss and are able to benefit from rehabilitation is a personal matter and may be a matter of days, months, or even years. In many cases, individuals who are slow to accept their prognosis will benefit from speaking to others who have gone through similar experiences or from discussing the situation with a professional counselor. For elders, the diagnosis of irreversible vision loss often heightens their awareness of failing physical abilities that accompany the aging process (Ainlay: 1989). In addition, vision loss affects the ability to follow instructions for taking medications; often causes falls; and results in many automobile accidents.

The role of professional service providers may be crucial in determining the individual's responses to the prognosis of diminished vision. Professionals who display an understanding of the problem and who are knowledgeable about the wide range of rehabilitation services may be the determining factor in the acceptance of vision loss and, ultimately, adjustment.

Social stigma associated with disabilities in general, and vision loss in particular, are difficult to overcome. Professionals who work with individuals who are visually impaired or blind can help to eliminate social stigma and negative stereotypes by facing the issue head on and providing knowledgeable referrals for patients and clients. All staff members who come in contact with people with vision loss should be knowledgeable about both the problems that vision loss causes as well as the range of help that is available. Knowledge of the available services may help to alleviate the fear that many professionals have about visual impairment and blindness and in turn will help them work more effectively with patients or clients.

BREAKING THE NEWS OF IRREVERSIBLE VISION LOSS

Breaking the news of irreversible vision loss (or of any irreversible impairment) is a difficult task. A frank yet sympathetic approach is best. Providing information about the many sources of assistance that can help the patient to continue functioning will make the task much easier and increase the patient's confidence in the service provider.

It is crucial that the ophthalmologist be the professional who explains the diagnosis, prognosis, and functional impairments to the patient or to the parents of a child who is visually impaired or blind. Passing this responsibility off to someone else in the ophthalmologist's office or leaving it to a social service professional suggests not only that the ophthalmologist is not concerned, but also deprives the patient and family of crucial medical information.

Ophthalmologists, optometrists, and other health care providers have the same fears about vision loss and blindness as other individuals. Because they encounter vision loss and blindness more frequently than most people, their fears may be greater unless they have learned about the many resources available to help people continue functioning. A good way for health care providers to learn about the resources available to people with vision loss is to invite a rehabilitation professional to visit their office. Health care professionals may also arrange to visit a rehabilitation agency to observe the rehabilitation process first hand. People who have successfully adjusted to vision loss are also good sources of information, and many are willing to talk about their experiences with rehabilitation.

A recent study indicated that ophthalmologists frequently underestimate patients' desire for information. In their study of patients with diabetic retinopathy and the ophthalmologists who treated them, Hopper and Fischbach (1989) discovered that most patients wanted to know everything about their condition and the results of their eye exam, and all patients wanted to know about the possibility of losing their vision. Their ophthalmologists, on the other hand, were far less likely to think that patients should know everything; only 38% thought that patients should know everything about their condition, the results of their eye exam, and the possibility of losing their vision. Although this study was small and confined to one large group practice, the findings parallel other studies that have found a discrepancy between the amount of information patients want and the amount of information physicians think is appropriate.

Greenblatt's (1991) study of individuals who had experienced vision loss within the four year period prior to the study found that many had not received the information they needed to obtain rehabilitation services. For example, most respondents indicated that their ophthalmologists had either not explained the definition of legal blindness at all or else they described the visual acuity criterion without mentioning the governmental benefits associated with legal blindness. Nor did ophthalmologists tell the respondents about the services available from the state agency that serves individuals who are visually impaired or blind. As a result, many respondents had no understanding of their entitlement to services.

Numerous studies (Jensen: 1981) have found that patients judge their physicians in large part on how caring they are. Patients who are dissatisfied with their physicians often cite inadequate explanations about the diagnosis and state that physicians ignore their questions. Thus the manner in which ophthalmologists break the news of irreversible vision loss may affect their own professional reputations; those who earn the reputation of being both frank and concerned will be more likely to have satisfied patients.

A discussion about the disease or condition that has caused the vision loss; the likely prognosis; its relationship to other health conditions; and possible treatments or ways of preventing further vision loss is crucial. Providing the patient with the opportunity to ask questions at the initial discussion, over the phone, and in follow-up appointments indicates that the ophthalmologist is concerned about the patient's adjustment. Ophthalmologists should avoid saying, "I'm sorry but there's nothing more I can do for you." Although there may be no medical or surgical intervention to restore vision to normal, a multitude of services exists to help people with vision loss.

It is important that patients know that they should return for ophthalmological examinations even when there is no cure for their current condition. If an ophthalmologist says there is "nothing more that can be done," some patients will construe this to mean that they should not seek future ophthalmological care. Patients with age-related macular degeneration who have been told by their ophthalmologists that nothing more can be done sometimes develop glaucoma or cataracts. Because their ophthalmologists said they could not offer any more help, the patients fail to schedule routine examinations and then lose part or all of their remaining peripheral vision due to other conditions.

Family members should usually be included in the discussion of vision loss and its implications, unless the patient requests otherwise. Patients and family members can rarely absorb all of the information they need to know at once; this is quite common at the time of diagnosis, when patients and family members may be in a state of emotional shock or trauma. Patients' needs for information will change during the adjustment process. Family members, especially those who live with the patient, should understand the limitations vision loss creates as well as the opportunities to receive services that help to overcome some of these limitations. It is important to remember that all patients and families are not alike. Some patients and families will request a great deal of information, while others will ask few questions. The ability to understand medical terms and procedures will also differ (Arkin: 1989).

For those individuals who have an eye disease or condition that causes progressive deterioration of vision, an explanation of the likely progression and early referrals may help facilitate the adjustment process. An honest assessment of the likely outcome in progressive diseases helps patients to plan their lives. For example, a person with retinitis pigmentosa or juvenile macular degeneration must be made aware that a career as an airplane pilot or a surgeon is unrealistic. On the other hand, with the proper adaptive equipment, people with these conditions may succeed in a wide variety of demanding professional careers. This information not only enables people with vision loss to plan their lives realistically, but it also helps them to adjust psychologically to their visual impairment.

Although it is important to stress the positive, giving false hope of a cure is misleading and may cause the patient to reject referrals for rehabilitation. Stating that research is being conducted to discover the cause, prevention, and cure of disease is important information, but the patient and family must not be led to believe that the cure is likely to be available in the near future if it is not. A poignant example of this well meaning but misguided type of information occurred when a prominent ophthalmologist told the mother of a boy with juvenile macular degeneration that research would lead to a cure for this disease. She in turn began making monthly calls to the research institute he had mentioned to ask if a cure had been found. Obviously, the way this information was presented and interpreted was counterproductive to the acceptance of the prognosis. Similarly, suggesting that someday there will be no need to use white canes or other devices that help people with vision loss to function is antithetical to the goals of rehabilitation, as it attaches a negative connotation to such devices. In fact, these devices have a very positive benefit for many individuals.

The prognosis of vision loss is usually difficult for the patient to accept. Such a response is normal. The professional's role at this point is to encourage follow-up conversations about the types of services that can help in the adjustment process.

The ophthalmologist should obtain information about the patient's current level of functioning. A good way to start a discussion is to ask, "What changes have occurred in your life since your vision has decreased?" Asking the patient about his or her major activities and interests (e.g., reading, writing, sewing, home-making, etc.) and whether the vision loss has interfered with these activities will provide information about the patient's specific needs regarding assistive devices and/or rehabilitation services.

The patient's ability to tend to practical needs such as independent travel and daily living skills will be affected by vision loss. Ask the patient about his or her living conditions. Does he or she live alone? If so, vision loss may be causing problems with home-making and self-care. Referral to a comprehensive rehabilitation agency that can assess the rehabilitation needs and provide training in daily living skills may be appropriate. Observe the patient's ability to get around in your office. If there are problems with mobility, a referral for orientation and mobility training is in order.

Ask about the patient's occupational situation. If he or she fears that vision loss may result in the loss of employment, make a referral to the state vocational rehabilitation agency for evaluation and training. Inform the patient about the many technological advances that have been made (such as computers with large print and/or speech output) that may enable a person who is visually impaired or blind to retain his or her job. (See Chapter 6, "Employment for People with Vision Loss")

Never assume that the patient is not in need of services because of advanced age. Only five percent of elders are institutionalized (Fowles: 1991). The remaining 95% live in their own homes or with relatives and need to perform common household activities and other tasks of daily living. Even an individual who can afford to hire staff to carry out household activities is likely to have experienced diminished self-esteem as a result of vision loss and should be offered the opportunity for rehabilitation services.

For those individuals with hereditary conditions, it is necessary to discuss the likelihood that they will pass on the condition to their offspring. In some instances, referral to a geneticist is appropriate.

Reinforcing the positive benefits of rehabilitation, suggesting self-help groups for those who want to learn more from others with vision loss, and displaying low vision aids in the office help the ophthalmologist in the delicate discussion that takes place. Ophthalmologists who follow these suggestions will receive much gratification from helping their patients.

THE MULTIDISCIPLINARY NATURE OF REHABILITATION

In order for people with vision loss to receive a coordinated plan for medical and rehabilitation care, the various professionals involved should meet to discuss the individual's case, including current health status, type and severity of the visual impairment, living arrangements, psychological status, and rehabilitation needs. Primary care providers, especially in cases where individuals have more than one impairment or medical condition, should be part of the multidisciplinary team that helps the individual to plan the rehabilitation course. The individual's own concerns and expressed needs are an important consideration in any discussion, whether or not the individual is present at the conference.

By establishing liaisons with rehabilitation professionals, health care providers can feel comfortable in knowing when and where to refer patients for appropriate services. Ophthalmologists often view low vision services as ancillary to their professional role; just as primary care physicians must be knowledgeable about appropriate rehabilitation for patients with a variety of disabilities and impairments, so too must ophthalmologists be familiar with the services available for patients with vision loss. Similarly, rehabilitation professionals must know how to ensure that their clients receive competent and adequate health care for medical problems that affect rehabilitation.

A recent study (Greenblatt: 1988b) of a national sample of practicing ophthalmologists found that those ophthalmologists who had received information more frequently from rehabilitation agencies were significantly more likely to refer for services and to carry out rehabilitation-oriented measures for patients on their own than were ophthalmologists who received this information less frequently. This finding suggests that professional service providers have the ability to influence each others' actions. In the case of providing services to people with vision loss, both health care providers and rehabilitation professionals should take advantage of this role as much as possible to ensure that individuals with vision loss receive optimal care.

Both health care providers and rehabilitation professionals should also be familiar with the advantages that self-help groups provide to many individuals. Although professionals should not be an integral part of self-help groups, they may play an important role in locating self-help groups for patients or clients or bringing together people with similar problems from within their practice (See Chapter 3, "Starting a Self-Help Group.").

Referral Guidelines for Health Care Professionals

Many individuals who have experienced vision loss may benefit from referrals to rehabilitation agencies, social workers, or peer support groups. Although not every individual needs or wants a referral, a good rule of thumb is to describe the various options. Individuals may not always accept the initial referral but may request further information at a later date.

If the patient is depressed, shocked, or simply unwilling to accept a referral, express your understanding of the difficulty in adjusting to the eye condition. Suggest the possibility of professional counseling or talking with other patients who have experienced similar vision problems (i.e., peer support groups). Medicare, Part B, reimburses for services provided by clinical social workers and psychologists. These professionals are required to consult with the individual's primary care physician unless specifically requested by the patient not to do so (Pampusch: 1990). If the patient rejects these suggestions but appears to be having problems managing everyday activities, schedule a follow-up appointment, making certain that the patient understands that the intent of the appointment is not for cure of the eye condition. If at the follow-up appointment, the patient still rejects all referrals, state that referrals for these services will be available if at some time in the future the patient wants them.

Many sources of assistance and information for individuals with vision loss as well as for professionals who work with these individuals are described in this manual. Sources are listed for special populations, by disease, and by function, such as reading or working. Many of these sources are national organizations that have local or regional offices, or they can make referrals to local agencies.

When making a referral, it is a good idea to provide a description of the services the agency provides. In addition, provide a letter to the agency documenting the patient's diagnosis, prognosis, and the reasons you have made the referral. Request that the agency report back to you concerning the patient's eligibility for services and the patient's progress or lack of progress. For a guide to the various professionals who are part of the rehabilitation team, see Weisse (1989).

Many individuals will benefit from the services of an orientation and mobility instructor. This rehabilitation professional provides instruction in safe travel techniques in the areas frequented by the individual in his or her neighborhood and at the workplace. Training in the use of a white cane increases the likelihood that travel will be safe and also alerts both pedestrians and drivers to the presence of someone who is visually impaired or blind. Professional service providers should encourage the use of the white cane, emphasizing its benefits and downplaying the social stigma sometimes attached to it. Referrals to guide dog training schools are another option for individuals who are visually impaired or blind; individuals considering a guide dog should be provided with information about the advantages and disadvantages of canes versus dogs.

Locating Services in Your Area

Once contacts have been made with one or two local rehabilitation agencies, health care providers will have the opportunity to learn about the variety of services that exist in their area. Although services are more plentiful in urban areas than in rural areas, information and referral networks can guide health care providers to the closest services. All states and provinces have agencies that provide rehabilitation services to eligible citizens, geographical location notwithstanding. In many instances, rehabilitation teachers and orientation and mobility instructors travel to the homes of people with vision loss to provide instruction.

If you have difficulty locating an agency in your area, contact the state agency that serves visually impaired and blind individuals. In some instances, this agency is an independent state agency and in other instances it is located within a state department of vocational rehabilitation, department of education, or department of labor. (See Appendix A for the address and telephone number of your state agency.) Although most states require that individuals be legally blind in order to qualify for services, individuals who are not legally blind may be referred to a private rehabilitation agency or a private practitioner, such as an ophthalmologist or optometrist who operates a low vision service; a rehabilitation teacher; or an orientation and mobility instructor.

Elders who have experienced vision loss but who are not legally blind may be eligible for services from a state department on aging or elder affairs or an area agency on aging (See Chapter 5, "Special Population Groups," Elders). Veterans with vision loss are eligible for services from VA Medical Centers throughout the country (See Chapter 5, "Special Population Groups," Veterans).

Other sources of information about local services for people with vision loss include the information service of the United Way; directories of local services available in the reference section of public libraries; senior centers; geriatric and ophthalmology departments of hospitals and medical schools; and schools of optometry.

If the Patient Is Legally Blind

In the U.S., individuals are considered to be legally blind if they have a visual acuity of 20/200 or worse in the better eye with all possible correction or a field restriction of 20 degrees diameter or less in the better eye. Most individuals who are legally blind retain some useful vision and should be encouraged to use it to the maximum extent possible. The classification of legal blindness entitles U.S. citizens to tax benefits as well as rehabilitation services provided by state governments. Definitions of legal blindness vary in other countries.

In many states, ophthalmologists and optometrists are required to register individuals who are "legally blind" with the state agency responsible for serving visually impaired and blind individuals. Every state has a public agency, often a Commission for the Blind, that serves this function. (See "Appendix A: State Agencies for Individuals Who Are Visually Impaired or Blind.")

Many professionals hesitate to inform patients about legal blindness because of the stigma attached to the word "blind." A frank discussion of visual functioning and an explanation that legal blindness is a categorization that entitles individuals to certain government benefits usually helps people overcome their fear of the word "blind." Explain that many agencies that have the word "blind" in their names serve individuals with varying degrees of visual impairment and that the agency's name should not be a deterrent to seeking services. The professional's understanding of the term legal blindness and an accurate explanation to the patient may have a major impact on the individual's willingness to accept services from rehabilitation professionals.

Referral Guidelines for Rehabilitation Professionals and Social Workers

Many of the suggestions made above for health care professionals are applicable to rehabilitation professionals and social workers when determining if additional referrals are necessary for individuals with vision loss. It is sometimes necessary to make a referral to ophthalmologists or optometrists for medical intervention or for the prescription of optical aids. Just as medical professionals should provide detailed information when making a referral for rehabilitation or social work services, rehabilitation professionals should provide detailed information about the individual when they make a referral to medical professionals. Always request that the health professional report back to you concerning findings and treatments for the individual who was referred. If your agency has a form for this purpose, include one with your letter of referral.

Reporting Back to the Health Care Professional

When you have received a referral from an ophthalmologist, optometrist, or an allied health professional, always report back to the referral source indicating what services have been provided to the individual who was referred. Send the medical professional information about the services your agency provides and add his or her name to the mailing list your agency uses for newsletters and to announce new services.

If the Client is Legally Blind

Individuals who are "legally blind" qualify for financial or other government services, yet many individuals who qualify are not aware of these benefits and have not been registered as "legally blind." If you believe that an individual you serve falls into this category, suggest that the individual visit an ophthalmologist or optometrist to determine the individual's acuity and field of vision. Discuss the meaning of the term "legally blind" with the individual and

Illustration 1

Reporting Legal Blindness

In states which do not have <u>Legal Blindness Report Forms</u>, use the following format when referring a patient for services.

Jane Smith, M.D.
345 Main St.
Anytown, MD

"This is to certify that <u>(patient's name)</u> is legally blind for income tax purposes. I examined <u>(patient's name)</u> on <u>(date)</u> and have diagnosed his/her eye condition as _____.

<u>(patient's name)</u>'s acuity is _____ O.S.; _____ O.D.; and his/her field is _____.

_____
Signature, Title

Be sure to tell the patient that he or she will be registered with the state agency. It is essential that patients hear directly from the ophthalmologist that they are "legally blind."

if necessary, phone the ophthalmologist or optometrist to discuss the individual's situation and his or her understanding of the term "legally blind." Suggest a meeting with the individual ophthalmologist or optometrist so that you can discuss the benefits that are available to patients who are registered as legally blind.

Over half of the states in the U.S. maintain registers of legal blindness (De Santis and Schein: 1986). In some states, the registration of individuals who are legally blind is required and in others it is voluntary. Check with the state agency that serves individuals who are visually impaired or blind to determine the proper procedures in your state.

HELPING PATIENTS OR CLIENTS ADJUST TO VISION LOSS

There are many ways that professionals can help people adjust to vision loss, in addition to referring for counseling or providing rehabilitation services. Included are making your own office environment comfortable for people with vision loss and learning some simple techniques to help individuals with vision loss move around your office safely and comfortably.

The Office Environment

The office setting may be made more comfortable for the patient or client without great effort or expense. Simple modifications will result in less anxiety for people with vision loss, and staff members will be less concerned about them falling or bumping into objects. Two obvious examples are providing good lighting and eliminating all possible sources of glare. The Americans with Disabilities Act, passed in July, 1990, requires that public accommodations, businesses, and services be accessible to individuals with disabilities. Public accommodations are broadly defined to include professional service providers' offices. After January 26, 1993, most new construction for public accommodations must be accessible to individuals with disabilities.

When moving to a new office, select a building with well-lighted hallways and accessible entries. Many people with vision loss also have other disabilities, and some may use walkers, canes, or wheelchairs for mobility. Building corridors and aisles within the office should be wide enough to accommodate these mobility aids and should not have clutter or projecting objects.

When designing or remodeling an office, the needs of people with vision loss should be a major concern. Contrasting colors should be used for carpeting, furniture, and walls. Yellow tape or painted stripes on the edge of steps enable people with vision loss to navigate the steps safely and feel more comfortable.

20

Intake forms and other forms for the patient or client to fill out should be made available in LARGE PRINT. Signs in the office should have large letters and good contrast. Several companies produce low vision acuity charts, which can help the patient achieve a certain amount of success in reading the letters and therefore provide encouragement. If there is a public telephone in the office, LARGE PRINT numerals will provide access for people who are visually impaired.

When entering a room, always introduce yourself by name and shake the person's hand; even if the person is unable to see your hand, he or she will probably extend a hand in greeting. While shaking hands is common etiquette, it also serves to make contact with the individual who may not be able to make eye contact due to vision loss. Entering a room quietly without introducing your presence can unpleasantly surprise a person who cannot see you. Similarly, you should always announce when you are leaving a room.

Providing Appropriate Literature

Literature that is distributed regarding the disease process and services available to people with vision loss should be made available in LARGE PRINT or on audiocassette. (Resources for Rehabilitation produces the "Living with Low Vision Series" of LARGE PRINT publications for this purpose. See references in appropriate chapters throughout this book and an order form on last page of this book.) Providing literature for the waiting room in LARGE PRINT also makes the person with vision loss and his or her family feel welcome. Waiting room subscriptions to LARGE PRINT publications such as the "Reader's Digest" and the "New York Times Large Type Weekly" inform individuals about periodicals available in this format.

Sighted Guide Technique

Health care providers, rehabilitation professionals, and all staff who work in senior citizen centers should be familiar with sighted guide technique. People with vision loss should never be pushed or pulled. Such an awkward method causes anxiety and places the person with vision loss in an unsafe position. Not all people with vision loss need help with travel. Some people with central vision loss are able to navigate without any assistance as are some people with moderate peripheral vision loss. The first step, therefore, is to always ask the person whether he or she needs assistance.

If the person indicates that assistance is needed, the sighted person should offer the person with vision loss his or her arm to hold just above the elbow and walk slightly ahead. By walking ahead of the person with vision loss, the sighted guide provides information about what is to come. For example, when the guide steps down a curb from the sidewalk to the street, the person with vision loss will feel that movement. Even people who have adjusted to their vision loss and are comfortable getting around on their own will appreciate a sighted guide in unfamiliar settings. In addition, mentioning the approach to a flight of steps or the entry onto an escalator or elevator provides the person with vision loss with additional important information. When giving directions, never say "over here" or "over there." Use specific words such as "left" and "right."

Call a local private or public rehabilitation agency which serves individuals who are visually impaired or blind to arrange a brief lesson in this technique. A request for training in sighted guide technique may also open the door to additional interactions with rehabilitation professionals.

LAWS AFFECTING PEOPLE WITH VISION LOSS

The number of laws affecting people with vision loss and other disabilities has grown rapidly in recent years; they cover a wide range of issues, including health care, financial benefits, housing, rehabilitation, civil rights, transportation, access to public buildings, and employment. Professional service providers must understand these laws in order to ensure that their patients and clients receive all the appropriate benefits and services that are available.

In July, 1990, the *Americans with Disabilities Act* (ADA) was passed (P.L. 101-336). Considered the most important civil rights legislation in recent years, the ADA defines an individual with a disability as a person who has a physical or mental impairment that substantially limits one or more major activities; someone who has had such an impairment; or someone who is regarded as having such an impairment. The ADA increases the steps employers must take to accommodate employees with disabilities (See Chapter 6, "Employment for People with Vision Loss" for more detailed information on this portion of the ADA); prohibits discrimination by public entities (i.e., local and state governments) in providing services and benefits to individuals with disabilities; and requires that public accommodations, businesses, and services be accessible to individuals with disabilities. Public accommodations are broadly defined to include places such as hotels and motels, theatres, museums, schools, shopping centers and stores, banks, restaurants, and professionals' offices.

Enforcement of the ADA is assigned to a variety of federal agencies, including the Department of Justice, the Architectural and Transportation Barriers Compliance Board, the Department of Transportation, and the Equal Employment Opportunity Commission (See "ORGANIZATIONS" section below). Copies of the ADA are available from Senators and Representatives. In addition, both public agencies and many private agencies that work with individuals who are visually impaired or blind have copies of the ADA available in special formats such as LARGE PRINT, audiocassette, and braille.

The *Rehabilitation Act of 1973* (P.L. 93-112) and its amendments are the centerpieces of federal law related to rehabilitation. Under this law, each state receives federal funding for providing rehabilitation services, after submitting a vocational rehabilitation plan to the

Rehabilitation Services Administration. Originally designed to help individuals with disabilities obtain jobs, vocational rehabilitation services are now more broadly defined. *Comprehensive Services for Independent Living* (P.L. 95-602) expanded rehabilitation services to individuals with severe disabilities, regardless of their vocational potential, making services available to many people who are no longer in the work force. The act defines services as any "service that will enhance the ability of a handicapped individual to live independently or function within his family and community..." These services may include counseling, job placement, housing, funds to make the home accessible, funds for prosthetic devices, attendant care, and recreational activities. The Civil Rights Division within the Department of Justice enforces the provisions of the Rehabilitation Act. The *Client Assistance Program* authorizes states to inform clients and other persons with disabilities about all benefits available under the Act and to assist them in obtaining all remedies due under the law (P.L. 98-221). Numerous additional provisions of this act are described in subsequent chapters of this book (See, for example, Chapter 5, "Special Population Groups," Children and Adolescents and Chapter 6, "Employment for People with Vision Loss.")

Supplementary Security Income (SSI) is a federal minimum income maintenance program for elders and individuals who are blind or disabled and who meet a test of financial need. Individuals need not have worked in order to qualify for SSI benefits.

Monthly *Social Security Disability Insurance* (SSDI) benefits are available to individuals who are disabled and their dependents. To be eligible, individuals must have paid Social Security taxes for a specified number of quarters (dependent upon the applicant's age); must not be working; and must be declared medically disabled by the state disability determination service or through an appeals process. Individuals who are legally blind and age 55 to 65 may receive monthly benefits if they are unable to carry out the work (or similar work) that they did before age 55 or becoming blind, whichever is later. Social Security disability benefits are not retroactive, so it is important to apply for them immediately after becoming legally blind.

Individuals who have received SSDI for two consecutive years are eligible for *Medicare*, a federal health insurance program, which may cover some of the necessary out-patient therapy or supplies discussed in this book. However, Medicare does not cover eyeglasses (except following cataract surgery), low vision aids, or hearing aids.

Medicaid is a joint federal/state health insurance plan for individuals who are considered financially needy (i.e., recipients of financial benefits from governmental assistance programs such as Aid to Families with Dependent Children or Supplemental Security Income). While federal law requires that each state cover hospital services, skilled nursing facility services, physician and home health care services, and diagnostic and screening services, states have great discretion in other areas. Payments for prosthetics and rehabilitation equipment vary by state.

Under amendments to the *Housing and Community Development Act of 1987* (P.L. 100-242), the Department of Housing and Urban Development provides direct loans for the development of projects for elders and individuals with disabilities. These developments may consist of apartments or group homes for up to 15 residents. The *Fair Housing Amendments Act of 1988* (P.L. 100-430) requires that multifamily dwellings designed for first occupancy after March 13, 1991 be accessible to individuals with disabilities. In addition, HUD has established programs to house individuals with disabilities who are homeless.

The federal government allows an extra personal exemption on federal income tax for individuals who are legally blind and do not itemize deductions; an extra standard deduction is allowed for those individuals who itemize deductions. Individuals who itemize their deductions may also take miscellaneous deductions (Impairment-Related Work Expenses) for expenditures such as readers and adapted computer hardware and software.

Deductible medical and dental expenses which exceed 7.5% of an individual's adjusted gross income may include special medications such as insulin and other special items such as guide dogs or other animals used by persons who are visually impaired, blind, or deaf. Some states allow extra personal exemptions for legal blindness on state income tax as well.

All states and many local governments have adopted their own laws regarding accessibility. Information about these laws may be obtained from the state or local office serving people with disabilities.

Some lawyers specialize in the legal needs of people with disabilities. The local bar association referral service or a law school can provide the names of specialists.

CONCLUSION

There are many ways that service providers can help people with vision loss continue functioning independently. These range from providing adequate information about the condition, its functional implications, and the prognosis, to modifying the office environment. Understanding the psychological responses to vision loss; making referrals for appropriate services; keeping abreast of benefits available under federal and state laws; and keeping in contact with other members of the rehabilitation team are all vital elements in helping people with vision loss.

References

Ainlay, Stephen C.
1989 Day Brought Back My Night: Aging and New Vision Loss New York, NY: Routledge

Arkin, Elaine Bratic
1989 <u>Making Health Communication Programs Work</u> Washington, DC: National Institutes of Health, Office of Cancer Communications, NIH Publication No. 89-1493

DeSantis, Vito and Jerome Schein
1986 "Blindness Statistics: Blindness Registers in the United States" <u>Journal of Visual Impairment and Blindness</u> 80(Feb):570-572

Fowles, D.
1991 <u>A Profile of Older Americans 1991</u> Washington, D.C.: American Association of Retired People

Greenblatt, Susan L.
1991   "What People with Vision Loss Need to Know" pp. 7-20 in Susan L. Greenblatt (ed.) <u>Meeting the Needs of People with Vision Loss: A Multidisciplinary Perspective</u> Lexington, MA: Resources for Rehabilitation
1988a   "Teaching Ophthalmology Residents About Rehabilitation" <u>Ophthalmology</u> 95:10:1468-1472
1988b   "Physicians and Chronic Impairment: A Study of Ophthalmologists' Interactions with Visually Impaired and Blind Patients" <u>Social Science and Medicine</u> 26:4 393-399

Hopper, Susan V. and Ruth L. Fischbach
1989 "Patient-Physician Communication When Blindness Threatens" <u>Patient Education and Counseling</u> 14:69-79

Hulnick, Mary R. and H. Ronald Hulnick
1989 "Life's Challenges: Curse or Opportunity? Counseling Families of Persons with Disabilities" <u>Journal of Counseling and Development</u> 68:166-170

Jensen, Peter S.
1981 "The Doctor-Patient Relationship: Headed for Impasse or Improvement?" <u>Annals of Internal Medicine</u> 95:769-771

National Center for Health Statistics
1989 "Practice Patterns of the Office-Based Ophthalmologist" National Ambulatory Medical Care Survey, 1985 <u>Advance data</u> number 162 Hyattsville, MD: Department of Health and Human Services, DHHS Publication (PHS) 89-1250
1981 <u>Prevalence of Selected Impairments: United States 1977</u> Department of Health and Human Services, Vital and Health Statistics, series 10, # 134) Hyattsville, MD: DHHS publication (PHS) 81-1562

Pampusch, Amy
1990 "Medicare to Cover Clinical Social Work," <u>Senior Patient</u> 2(5):24

Schappert, Susan M.
1992 "National Ambulatory Medical Carey Survey: 1990 Summary" <u>Advance Data</u> April 30, number 213, Hyattsville, MD: National Center for Health Statistics

Sommer, Alfred, James M. Tielsch, Joanne Katz, Harry A. Quigley, John D. Gottsch, Jonathan C. Javitt, James F. Martone, Richard M. Royall, Kathe Witt, and Sandi Ezrine
1991 "Racial Differences in the Cause-Specific Prevalence of Blindness in East Baltimore <u>New England Journal of Medicine</u> 325(November 14):1412-7

Statistics Canada
1988 <u>The Health and Activity Limitation Survey: User's Guide</u>, Ottawa, Canada

Tielsch, James M., Alfred Sommer, Kathe Witt, Joanne Katz, and Richard M. Royall
1990 "Blindness and Visual Impairment in an American Population" <u>Archives of Ophthalmology</u> 108(February):286-290

Weisse, Fran A.
1989 "Making Referrals for Rehabilitation Services" pp. 56-71 in Susan L. Greenblatt (ed.) <u>Providing Services for People with Vision Loss: A Multidisciplinary Perspective</u> Lexington, MA: Resources for Rehabilitation

Chapter 2

SOURCES OF GENERAL INFORMATION ON VISION LOSS

PROFESSIONAL ORGANIZATIONS

(In the listings below, telephone numbers have symbols V for voice and TT for text telephone where organizations have published this information.)

American Academy of Ophthalmology (AAO)
655 Beach Street
San Francisco, CA 94109
(415) 561-8500   FAX (415) 561-8533

Professional membership organization that provides information on common eye diseases. One of its standing committees is composed of individuals with a special interest in low vision and rehabilitation. Sponsors the National Eye Care Project, which makes referrals to an ophthalmologist for individuals 65 years and older who do not currently have an ophthalmologist [(800) 222-3937].

American Optometric Association (AOA)
243 North Lindbergh Boulevard
St. Louis, MO 63141
(314) 991-4100

Professional membership organization. Provides information on the most common eye diseases and conditions to its members and the public. Special membership in low vision section, which promotes low vision care services and serves as a source of information to professionals and the public. Produces "A Gift of Sight," a videotape describing low vision and services available to patients. $35.00

Association for Education and Rehabilitation of the Blind and Visually Impaired (AER)
206 North Washington Street
Alexandria, VA 22314
(703) 548-1884

Membership organization of rehabilitation counselors and teachers, orientation and mobility instructors, special educators, psychologists, health care providers, and other professionals with an interest in visual impairment. Publishes newsletter, "AER Report;" holds regional and international meetings; sets standards for certification. Membership benefits include subscription to "RE:view," quarterly journal.

Canadian Rehabilitation Council for the Disabled (CRCD)
45 Sheppard Avenue East, Suite 801
Toronto, Ontario M2N 5W9 Canada
(416) 250-7490 (V/TT)   FAX (416) 229-1371

A federation of regional and provincial groups that serve people with disabilities in Canada. Operates an information service and publishes a newsletter, "Access" and "Rehabilitation Digest" a quarterly journal with news about rehabilitation in Canada.

National Rehabilitation Association (NRA)
1910 Association Drive, Suite 205
Reston, VA 22091-1502
(703) 715-9090   (703) 715-9209 (TT)   FAX 715-1058

Membership organization for professionals who work in the field of rehabilitation. Holds annual training conference. Membership benefits include "Journal of Rehabilitation" and "NRA Newsletter."

Resources for Rehabilitation
33 Bedford Street, Suite 19A
Lexington, MA 02173
(617) 862-6455   FAX (617) 861-7517

Conducts training programs for health, social service, rehabilitation professionals, and employers on a contractual basis or for an admission fee. Write or call to arrange special programs at your institution or to be notified about programs in your area. Publishes the "Living with Low Vision Series" which includes LARGE PRINT (18 point bold) publications designed for distribution by professionals to people with vision loss, "Meeting the Needs of People with Vision Loss: A Multidisciplinary Perspective," and "Providing Services for People with Vision Loss: A Multidisciplinary Perspective." See pages 255 to 256 of this book for descriptions and prices.

Electronic Industries Foundation (EIF)
919 18th Street, Suite 900
Washington, DC 20006
(202) 955-5810   (202) 955-5836 (TT)   FAX (202) 955-5837

Studies policy issues to further the appropriate use of technology by individuals with disabilities (i.e. funding strategies). Conducts research aimed at expediting the dissemination of knowledge and technology transfer that can help people with disabilities.

Institute for Scientific Research (ISR)
33 Bedford Street, Suite 19A
Lexington, MA 02173
(617) 862-6455   FAX (617) 861-7517

Conducts research on the sociological aspects of vision loss and other disabilities and rehabilitation. Conducts evaluations of programs designed to train professionals and to rehabilitate individuals with vision loss and other disabilities.

National Eye Institute (NEI)
Building 31, Room 6A32
Bethesda, MD 20892
(301) 496-5248

Conducts basic, epidemiological, and clinical research into the causes and cures of eye diseases. Reports on research through "Clinical Trials Supported by the National Eye Institute," available from the Scientific Reporting Section. Patients are recruited for a variety of clinical studies supported by NEI; to obtain information, contact NEI directly. Ophthalmology (published by the American Academy of Ophthalmology and available from J. B. Lippincott Company, East Washington Square, Philadelphia, PA 800-638-3030) publishes a list of studies that are currently recruiting patients and the phone numbers for the Study Center Offices.

National Institute on Disability and Rehabilitation Research (NIDRR)
U.S. Department of Education
400 Maryland Avenue, SW
Washington, DC 20202
(202) 205-8134   (202) 205-5479 (TT)   FAX (202) 205-8515
(202) 205-8207 client information recording

A federal organization that funds research into various aspects of disability and rehabilitation, including the development of aids and devices that help people with disabilities to function independently; demographic analyses; and social science research. Grant programs are announced in the "Federal Register" or information may be obtained by phoning NIDRR's client information recording listed above.

National Research Council (NRC)
Committee on Vision
2101 Constitution Avenue, NW
Washington, DC 20418
(202) 334-2000

A standing committee of the NRC's Commission on Behavioral and Social Sciences and Education that investigates scientific issues related to vision. Holds scientific meetings and produces publications.

Rehabilitation Engineering Center of the Smith Kettlewell Eye Research Institute
2232 Webster Street
San Francisco, CA 94115
(415) 561-1619   FAX (415) 561-1610

A federally funded center that develops and tests new technology for individuals who are visually impaired, blind, or deaf-blind.

Research to Prevent Blindness (RPB)
598 Madison Avenue
New York, NY 10022
(212) 752-4333

Funds scientists and ophthalmologists to conduct research, establish research centers, and purchase equipment for laboratories. Sponsors conferences and distributes scientific publications.

Schepens Eye Research Institute
20 Staniford Street
Boston, MA 02114
(617) 742-3140

Conducts research in biomedical physics, clinical research, cornea, neuroscience, ocular ophthalmological pharmacology, physiological optics, and vitreo-retinal biochemistry and cell biology. Newsletter, "Sundial," FREE.

Social Research Department
American Foundation for the Blind
15 West 16th Street
New York, NY 10011
(212) 620-2140

Conducts sociological and statistical research in the field of visual impairment and blindness.

U.S. Department of Veteran Affairs (VA)

The VA's Blind Rehabilitation Centers conduct research on low vision training, low vision aids, computer aids, psychosocial aspects of visual impairment, and mobility aids. For locations of Blind Rehabilitation Centers, see Chapter 5, "Special Population Groups," Veterans.

World Rehabilitation Fund
International Exchange of Experts and Information in Rehabilitation
Institute on Disability
University of New Hampshire
6 Hood House
Durham, NH 03824-3577
(603) 862-4767   FAX (603) 862-4217

Administers a federally funded program that provides fellowships for researchers to travel abroad to study rehabilitation practices, policies, and research in other countries. Disseminates research finding through monographs, workshops, and conferences.

PROFESSIONAL PUBLICATIONS

The following bibliography lists major publications in the area of vision loss and disability. It is not meant to be comprehensive, but rather to provide the reader with a starting point for seeking out general references in the field. Additional professional references are provided in succeeding chapters. Some books listed below may be out of print but have been included because they are considered to be classics. These books are usually available in academic libraries.

Books and Articles

Bauman, Mary K.
1976 Blindness, Visual Impairment, Deaf-Blindness: Annotated Listing of the Literature, 1953-75 Philadelphia, PA: Temple University Press

Berkowitz, Edward D.
1987 <u>Disabled Policy: America's Programs for the Handicapped</u> New York, NY: Cambridge University Press

Carroll, Thomas J.
1961 <u>Blindness: What It Is, What It Does, and How to Live with It</u> Boston, MA: Little Brown

Cholden, Louis
1959 <u>A Psychiatrist Looks at Blindness</u> New York, NY: American Foundation for the Blind

Conyers, Maria
1992 <u>Vision for the Future: Meeting the Challenge of Sight Loss</u> London, England: Jessica Kingsley (available from Taylor and Francis, 1900 Frost Road, Suite 101, Bristol, PA 19007)

Demer, Joseph L., Franklin I. Porter, Jefim Goldberg, Herman A. Jenkins, Kim Schmidt, and Imogen Ulricht
1989 "Predictors of Functional Success in Telescopic Spectacle Use by Low Vision Patients" <u>Investigative Ophthalmology and Visual Science</u> 30:1660-1665

DeSantis, Vito and Jerome Schein
1986 "Blindness Statistics: Blindness Registers in the United States" <u>Journal of Visual Impairment and Blindness</u> 80:570-572

Edwards, Laura A. (ed.)
1986 <u>Rehabilitation of Low Vision Individuals</u> National Rehabilitation Information Center, 8455 Colesville Road, Suite 935, Silver Spring, MD 20910-3319

Emerson, Donna L.
1981 "Facing Loss of Vision: The Response of Adults to Visual Impairment" <u>Journal of Visual Impairment and Blindness</u> 75:41-45

Evans, Lawrence S.
1989 "Operating a Low Vision Aids Service" pp. 39-55 in Susan L. Greenblatt (ed.) <u>Providing Services for People with Vision Loss: A Multidisciplinary Perspective</u> Lexington, MA: Resources for Rehabilitation

Fatt, Helene V., John R. Griffin, and William M. Lyle
1992 <u>Genetics for Primary Eye Care Practitioners</u>, second edition, Stoneham, MA: Butterworth

Faye, Eleanor E.
1984 <u>Clinical Low Vision</u> Boston, MA: Little Brown & Co.

Fichten, Catherine S., Gabrielle Goodrick, Rhonda Amsel, and Susanne Wicks McKenzie
1991 "Reactions Toward Dating Peers with Visual Impairments" <u>Rehabilitation Psychology</u>
    36(3):163-178

Fletcher, Donald C.
1989 "Vision Loss: The Ophthalmologist's Perspective" pp. 16-24 in Susan L. Greenblatt
    (ed.) <u>Providing Services for People with Vision Loss: A Multidisciplinary Perspective</u>
    Lexington, MA: Resources for Rehabilitation

Fonda, Gerald E.
1991 "Designing Half-eye Binocular Spectacle Magnifiers" <u>Survey of Ophthalmology</u>
    36(September/October):149-54
1984 <u>Management of Low Vision</u> New York, NY: Grune-Stratton, Inc.

Foxall, Martha J., Cecilia R. Barron, Kathleen Von Dollen, Patricia A. Jones, and Kelly A.
Shull
1992 "Predictors of Loneliness in Low Vision Adults" <u>Western Journal of Nursing Research</u>
    4(1): 86-99

Freeman, Paul R. and Randall T. Jose
1991 <u>The Art and Practice of Low Vision</u> Stoneham, MA: Butterworth

Goodman, William
1989 <u>Mobility Training for People with Disabilities: Children and Adults with Physical,</u>
    <u>Mental, Visual and Hearing Impairments Can Learn to Travel</u> Springfield, IL: Charles
    C. Thomas

Goodrich, Gregory L. and Randall T. Jose
1992 <u>Low Vision: The Reference</u> New York, NY: Lighthouse National Center for Vision and
    Aging

Greenblatt, Susan L.
1991 <u>Meeting the Needs of People with Vision Loss: A Multidisciplinary Perspective</u>
    Lexington, MA: Resources for Rehabilitation
1990 "Training Ophthalmology Residents to Treat Patients with Vision Loss: Results of a
    Demonstration Program" <u>Ophthalmology</u> 97:1:138-143
1989 <u>Providing Services for People with Vision Loss: A Multidisciplinary Perspective</u>
    Lexington, MA: Resources for Rehabilitation
1988 "Teaching Ophthalmology Residents About Rehabilitation" <u>Ophthalmology</u> 95:10:1468-
    1472
1988 "Physicians and Chronic Impairment: A Study of Ophthalmologists' Interactions with
    Visually Impaired and Blind Patients" <u>Social Science and Medicine</u> 26:393-399

Hoehne, Charles. W., John G. Cull, and Richard E. Hardy (eds.)
1980 <u>Ophthalmological Considerations in the Rehabilitation of the Blind</u> Springfield, IL: Charles C. Thomas

Hollins, Mark
1989 <u>Understanding Blindness: A Multidisciplinary Approach</u> Hillsdale, NJ: Lawrence Erlbaum Associates

Hoover, Richard E.
1967 "The Ophthalmologist's Role in New Rehabilitation Patterns" <u>Transactions of the American Ophthalmology Society</u> 65:471-492

Jose, Randall T.
1983 <u>Understanding Low Vision</u> New York, NY: American Foundation for the Blind

Kirchner, Corinne
1989 <u>Data on Blindness and Visual Impairment in the U.S.</u> New York, NY: American Foundation for the Blind

Koestler, Frances A.
1976 <u>The Unseen Minority: A Social History of Blindness in the United States</u> New York, NY: American Foundation for the Blind

Maloff, Chalda and Susan Macduff Wood
1988 <u>Business and Social Etiquette with Disabled People: A Guide to Getting Along With Persons Who Have Impairments Of Mobility, Vision, Hearing, or Speech</u> Springfield, IL: Charles C. Thomas

McIlwaine, Gawn G., John A. Bell, and Gordon N. Dutton
1991 "Low Vision Aids Is our Service Cost Effective?" <u>Eye</u> 5:607-11

National Eye Institute
1987 <u>Vision Research - A National Plan</u> 1987 Evaluation and Update U.S. Department of Health and Human Services, Public Health Service, National Institutes of Health
1983 <u>Vision Research - A National Plan 1983-1987</u> U.S. Department of Health and Human Services, Public Health Service, National Institutes of Health

National Library Service for the Blind and Physically Handicapped
1991 <u>Disability Awareness and Changing Attitudes</u>
1990 <u>Building a Library Collection on Blindness and Physical Handicaps: Basic Materials and Resources</u> NLS, 1291 Taylor Street, NW, Washington, DC 20542

Organization for Social and Technical Innovations (OSTI)
1968 Blindness and Services to the Blind in the U.S.   Washington, D.C.: National Institute
    of Neurological Diseases and Blindness

Overbury, O., W. B. Jackson, and C. Hagenson
1987 "Factors Affecting the Successful Use of Low Vision Aids" Canadian Journal of
    Ophthalmology 22:205-207

Rehabilitation International
1989 Ethical Issues in Disability and Rehabilitation Rehabilitation International, 25 East 21st
    Street, New York, NY 10010

Research Grant Guides
1992 Handicapped Funding Directory Research Grant Guides, PO Box 1214, Loxahatchee,
    FL 33470

Ross, Caroline K., Joan A. Stelmack, Thomas R. Stelmack, and Melanie Fraim
1991 "Preliminary Examination of the Reliability and Relation to Clinical State of a Measure
    of Low Vision Patient Functional Status" Optometry and Vision Science 68(12):918-
    23

Sardegna, Jill and T. Otis Paul
1991 The Encyclopedia of Blindness and Visual Impairment New York, NY: Facts on File

Schein, Jerome D. and Vito J. DeSantis
1986 "Blindness Statistics: An Analysis of Operational Options" Journal of Visual Impairment
    and Blindness 80:517-522

Scott, Robert A.
1969 The Making of Blind Men New York, NY: Russell Sage Foundation
1967 "The Selection of Clients by Social Welfare Agencies: The Case of the Blind" Social
    Problems 14 (Winter): 248-257

Stubbins, Joseph (ed.)
1977 Social and Psychological Aspects of Disability: A Handbook for Practitioners
    Baltimore, MD: University Park Press

Tielsch, James, M. Alfred Sommer, Joanne Katz, Harry Quigley, Sandi Ezrine, and the
Baltimore Eye Survey Research Group
1991 "Socioeconomic Status and Visual Impairment Among Urban Americans" Archives of
    Ophthalmology 109(May):637-641

Turnbull, H.R., A.P. Turnbull, G.J. Bronicki, J.A. Summers, and C. Roeder-Gordon
1989 Disability and the Family: A Guide to Decisions for Adulthood Baltimore, MD: Paul H. Brookes

Tuttle, Dean W.
1984 Self-Esteem and Adjusting with Blindness: The Process of Responding to Life's Demands Springfield, IL: Charles C. Thomas

Uslan, Mark M., Everett W. Hill, and Alec F. Peck
1989 The Profession of Orientation and Mobility in the 1980s: The AFB Competency Study New York, NY: American Foundation for the Blind

Van Rens, G.H.M.B., R.J.M. Chmielowski, and W.A.J.G. Lemmens
1991 "Results Obtained with Low Vision Aids" Documenta Ophthalmologica 78:205-210

Vaughan, C. Edwin
1991 "The Social Basis of Conflict between Blind People and Agents of Rehabilitation" Disability, Handicap, and Society 6(3):203-17

Virtanen, Pekka and Leila Laatkainen
1991 "Primary Success with Low Vision Aids in Age-related Macular Degeneration" Acta Ophthalmologica 69:484-90

Wainapel, Stanley F.
1989 "Vision Loss: A Patient's Perspective" pp. 6-15 in Susan L. Greenblatt (ed.) Providing Services for People with Vision Loss: A Multidisciplinary Perspective Lexington, MA: Resources for Rehabilitation

Wainapel, Stanley F. and Marla Bernbaum
1986 "The Physician with Visual Impairment or Blindness" Archives of Ophthalmology, 104(Apr):498-502

Warnke, James W.
1989 "Mental Health Services: The Missing Link" pp. 72-83 in Susan L. Greenblatt (ed.) Providing Services for People with Vision Loss: A Multidisciplinary Perspective Lexington, MA: Resources for Rehabilitation

Welsh, Richard L. and Bruce B. Blasch
1980 Foundations of Orientation and Mobility New York, NY: American Foundation for the Blind

Woo, G.C., (ed.)
1986 Low Vision: Principles and Applications New York, NY: Springer Verlag

Wright, Tennyson J. and William G. Emener, (eds.)
1989 <u>Ethnic Minorities with Disabilities: An Annotated Bibliography of Rehabilitation Literature</u> Tampa, FL: Department of Rehabilitation Counseling, University of South Florida

Wulsin, Lawson R., Alan M. Jacobson, and Lawrence I. Rand
1991 "Psychosocial Correlates of Mild Visual Loss" <u>Psychosomatic Medicine</u> 53:109-17

Yuker, Harold E. (ed.)
1988 <u>Attitudes Toward Persons with Disabilities</u> New York, NY: Springer Publishing Company

Zimmerman, George J.
1992 "Orientation and Mobility Training" <u>Journal of Vocational Rehabilitation</u> 2(1)66-72

Journals

<u>American Rehabilitation</u>
Superintendent of Documents
U.S. Government Printing Office
Washington, DC 20402

Published by the Rehabilitation Services Administration of the U.S. Department of Education, this publication includes articles about developments in the field of rehabilitation, laws affecting rehabilitation, and news about publications. U.S., $5.00; foreign, $6.25.

<u>Disability Studies Quarterly</u>
Sociology Department
Brandeis University
Waltham, MA 02254
(617) 736-2645   FAX (617) 736-2653

Reports on recent research findings, upcoming meetings, grant solicitations. Book and audiovisual reviews. Individual subscription rate U.S., $20.00; Canada, $25.00.

<u>International Journal of Rehabilitation Research</u>
Journals, Chapman and Hall
20 West 35th Street
New York, NY 10001-2291

A quarterly journal with articles on research and practice written by professionals from a variety of disciplines in both developed and developing societies. U.S. and Canada, $80.00.

Journal of Rehabilitation
National Rehabilitation Association (NRA)
1910 Association Drive, Suite 205
Reston, VA 22091-1502
(703) 715-9090   (703) 715-9209 (TT)   FAX (703) 715-1058

A quarterly journal with articles by professionals from a variety of specialties within rehabilitation. U.S., $35.00; Canada, $40.00; foreign, $50.00.

Journal of Rehabilitation Research and Development
Office of Technology Transfer, VA Prosthetics R & D Center
103 South Gay Street
Baltimore, MD 21202
(410) 962-1800

A quarterly journal that includes articles on disability rehabilitation, sensory aids, gerontology, and other disabling conditions. Annual supplements provide research progress reports. Clinical supplements report on specific topics. FREE

Journal of Vision Rehabilitation
Media Productions & Marketing, Inc.
2440 O Street, Suite 202
Lincoln, NE 68510

A multidisciplinary journal published four times per year. $50.00

Journal of Visual Impairment and Blindness
American Foundation for the Blind (AFB)
15 West 16th Street
New York, NY 10011
(800) 232-5463   (212) 620-2000   FAX (212) 620-2105

A multidisciplinary journal for practitioners and researchers available in print, audiocassette, or braille. Published monthly, except July and August. $40.00

RE:view
Heldref Publications
1319 18th Street, NW, Department HS
Washington, DC 20036-1802
(800) 365-9753   (202) 296-6267   FAX (202) 296-5149

A quarterly journal with articles about services for children and adults who are visually impaired or blind. Individuals, $23.00; institutions, $45.00, foreign, add $10.00 for postage.

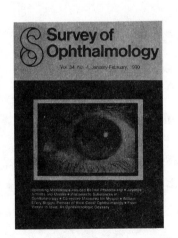

REFERRAL RESOURCES

Organizations

(In the listings below, telephone numbers have symbols V for voice and TT for text telephone where organizations have published this information.)

Alliance of Genetic Support Groups
35 Wisconsin Circle, Suite 440
Chevy Chase, MD 20815
(800) 336-4363   (301) 652-5553   FAX (301) 654-0171

Provides education and services to families and individuals affected by genetic disorders. Monthly news bulletin, "Alliance Alert." Membership, individuals, $15.00; organizations, $40.00.

American Council of the Blind (ACB)
1155 15th Street, NW, Suite 720
Washington, DC 20005
(800) 424-8666   (202) 467-5081   FAX (202) 467-5085

Membership organization with chapters in many states. Special interest groups such as blind parents, guide dog users, low vision, students, etc. Publishes the "Braille Forum," a bimonthly newsletter available in LARGE PRINT, audiocassette, and braille. Membership, $5.00.

American Foundation for the Blind (AFB)
15 West 16th Street
New York, NY 10011
(800) 232-5463   (212) 620-2000   FAX (212) 620-2105

An information clearinghouse on blindness and visual impairment. "Publications Catalog" and "AFB Products for People with Vision Problems," FREE.

Architectural and Transportation Barriers Compliance Board (ATBCB)
1331 F Street, NW, Suite 1000
Washington, DC 20004-1111
(800) 872-2253 (V/TT)   (202) 272-5434   (202) 272-5449 (TT)
FAX (202) 272-5447

A federal agency charged with developing standards for accessibility in federal facilities, public accommodations, and transportation facilities as required by the Americans with Disabilities Act and other federal laws. Provides technical assistance, sponsors research, and distributes publications. Publishes a quarterly newsletter, "Access America." Publications available in standard print, LARGE PRINT, audiocassette, computer disk, and braille. FREE

Canadian National Institute for the Blind (CNIB)
National Office
1931 Bayview Avenue
Toronto, Ontario M4G 4C8 Canada
(416) 480-7580   FAX (416) 480-7677

CNIB provides services to Canadians with any degree of functional vision impairment. Operates resource centres and technology centres and provides special services for seniors, veterans, and people who are deaf-blind. Public information literature available. See Appendix B: Division Offices of the Canadian National Institute for the Blind.

Council of Citizens with Low Vision International (CCLVI)
5707 Brockton Drive, #302
Indianapolis, IN 46220-5481
(800) 733-2258   (317) 254-1185   FAX (317) 251-6588

Provides support, education, and advocacy. Publishes "CCLVI News," a quarterly newsletter available in LARGE PRINT and audiocassette. Membership, $5.00

Department of Health and Human Services
Office of Civil Rights
330 Independence Avenue, SW (Cohen Building)
Washington, DC 20201
(202) 619-0585   (202) 863-0101 (TT)   FAX (202) 619-3437

Responsible for enforcing laws and regulations that protect the rights of individuals seeking medical and social services in institutions that receive federal financial assistance. Individuals who feel their rights have been violated may file a complaint with one of the ten regional offices located throughout the country.

Department of Housing and Urban Development (HUD)
Office of Elderly and Assisted Housing
Washington, DC 20410
(202) 708-2866

Operates programs to make housing accessible, including loan and mortgage insurance for rehabilitation of single or multifamily units. FREE information kit.

Department of Justice
Civil Rights Division
PO Box 66118
Washington, DC 20035-6118
(202) 514-0301 (V)   (202) 514-0381 (TT)   (202) 514-0383 (TT)

Responsible for enforcing the Americans with Disabilities Act and sections 503 and 504 of the Rehabilitation Act. Copies of its regulations are available in standard print, LARGE PRINT, braille, computer disk, audiocassette, and on an electronic bulletin board, (202) 514-6193.

Equal Employment Opportunity Commission (EEOC)
1801 L Street, NW, 10th floor
Washington, DC 20507
Recorded messages in English and Spanish; order publications and forms to file complaints; and option to speak with an EEOC employee:
(800) 669-3362 for calls from touch tone phones
(800) 669-4000 for calls from rotary dial phones
(800) 800-3302 (TT)

Responsible for developing and enforcing regulations for the employment section of the ADA. Copies of its regulations are available in standard print, LARGE PRINT, audiocassette, computer disk, and braille.

National Association for Visually Handicapped (NAVH)
22 West 21st Street
New York, NY 10010
(212) 889-3141

Distributes LARGE PRINT books; sells low vision aids; and produces two LARGE PRINT newsletters, "Seeing Clearly," for adults, and "In Focus," for youth, both FREE. Membership, $35.00. FREE catalogue.

National Federation of the Blind (NFB)
1800 Johnson Street
Baltimore, MD 21230
(410) 659-9314   FAX (410) 685-5653

National membership organization with chapters in many states. Provides information about available services, laws, and evaluation of new technology. Special interest groups for students, parents of blind children, etc. Holds state and national annual conventions. Publishes the "Braille Monitor," a monthly magazine available in standard print, audiocassette, disc, and braille. $25.00 per year contribution requested.

National Library Service for the Blind and Physically Handicapped (NLS)
1291 Taylor Street, NW
Washington, DC 20542
(800) 424-8567 or 8572 (Reference Section)
(800) 424-9100 (to receive application)
(202) 707-5100   FAX (202) 707-0712

National library service that serves individuals in the U.S. and U.S. residents living abroad. Regional libraries in many states. Individuals must be unable to read standard print due to visual impairment or physical disability. "Facts: Books for Blind and Physically Handicapped Individuals" describes NLS programs and eligibility requirements. Order form lists general information brochures, magazines and newsletters, directories, reference circulars, and subject and reference bibliographies. "Talking Book Topics," published bimonthly, in LARGE PRINT, audiocassette, and disc, lists titles recently added to the national collection which are available through the network of regional libraries. All services and publications from NLS are FREE (See Chapter 7, "Special Reading Resources and Services.")

National Rehabilitation Information Center (NARIC)
8455 Colesville Road, Suite 935
Silver Spring, MD 20910-3319
(800) 346-2742   (301) 588-9284 (V/TT)

A center that responds to inquiries about disabilities and support services. Newsletter, "NARIC Quarterly," FREE.

National Society to Prevent Blindness (NSPB)
500 East Remington Road
Schaumburg, IL 60173
(800) 221-3004   (708) 843-2020   FAX (708) 843-8458

Sponsors vision screenings. Local and state affiliates. Publications related to diseases and eye injuries, including some in Spanish, Chinese, and Portuguese. FREE catalogue.

Office of Transportation Regulatory Affairs
Department of Transportation
400 Seventh Street, SW
Washington, DC 20590
(202) 366-9305   (202) 755-7687 (TT)

Responsible for developing regulations for transportation of individuals with disabilities required by the Rehabilitation Act and the Americans with Disabilities Act. Regulations available in standard print and audiocassette.

United Way/Centraide Canada
600-150 Kent
Ottawa, Ontario K1P 5P4 Canada
(613) 236-7041

United Way of America (UWA)
701 North Fairfax Street
Alexandria, VA 22314-2045
(703) 836-7100

An umbrella organization which links local human service organizations. Look in the phone book for the United Way in your area. National offices in the U.S. and Canada can direct you to the local UW which will provide referral to specific services in your community.

VISION Foundation, Inc.
818 Mt. Auburn Street
Watertown, MA 02172
(617) 926-4232   In MA, (800) 852-3029

Information center for individuals with sight loss. Publishes materials in LARGE PRINT and audiocassette, including the VISION Resource List (FREE) and "VISION Resource Update," a bimonthly resource newsletter (membership benefit). Membership, individuals, $20.00; seniors, $10.00; families, $30.00; organizations, $35.00.

Coping with the Diagnosis of Sight Loss
Resources for Rehabilitation
33 Bedford Street, Suite 19A
Lexington, MA 02173
(617) 862-6455   FAX (617) 861-7517

Three consumers discuss their reactions and experiences when told that they were losing their vision. Audiocassette, $12.00 plus $3.00 shipping and handling

The Encounter
Carmichael Audio-Video Duplication
5135 Leavenworth Street
Omaha, NE 68106

A videotape about interactions between people with normal vision and those who are blind produced by the Nebraska Department of Public Institutions. The tape uses humor to show how people who are blind are capable of independent activities; it also addresses education and employment opportunities. 11 minutes. VHS $8.50

The First Steps: How To Help People Who Are Losing Their Sight
Peninsula Center for the Blind
4151 Middlefield Road
Palo Alto, CA 94303
(415) 858-0202   In CA, from area code 408, (800) 660-2009

A booklet written to answer some of the initial questions and discuss some of the immediate reactions people have when blindness first occurs in a family. $8.25

If Blindness Strikes: Don't Strike Out
by Margaret Smith
Charles C. Thomas, Springfield, IL

Written by a rehabilitation counselor who is visually impaired, this book describes many adaptations and strategies for living with vision loss. $40.00. Also available on audiocassette on loan from the National Library Service for the Blind and Physically Handicapped regional libraries, RC 21060. To purchase two-track ($13.50) or four-track ($7.50) audiocassettes, contact Readings for the Blind, 29451 Greenfield Road, Suite 118, Southfield, MI 48076; (313) 557-7776.

Independent Living
Equal Opportunity Publications
44 Broadway
Greenlawn, NY 11740
(516) 261-9086

A magazine that addresses the needs of individuals with disabilities in everyday life, including careers and health care issues. FREE

Living with Low Vision: A Resource Guide for People with Sight Loss
Resources for Rehabilitation
33 Bedford Street, Suite 19A
Lexington, MA 02173
(617) 862-6455   FAX (617) 861-7517

A LARGE PRINT comprehensive directory that helps people with sight loss remain independent. Lists services and products that enable individuals to keep reading, working, and carrying out daily activities. Updated biennially. $35.00 plus $5.00 shipping and handling.

Living with Vision Loss
Canadian National Institute for the Blind (CNIB)
1931 Bayview Avenue
Toronto, Ontario M4G 4C8 Canada
(416) 480-7626   FAX (416) 480-7677

A videotape with information on causes of visual impairment and adaptations for everyday life including lighting, kitchen skills, and travel. 13 minutes. VHS or BETA, $45.00; 3/4 inch, $70.00; Canadian funds

Living with Vision Loss: A Handbook for Caregivers
Canadian National Institute for the Blind (CNIB)
Rehabilitation Department
1931 Bayview Avenue
Toronto, Ontario M4G 4C8 Canada
(416) 480-7626   FAX (416) 480-7677

Practical suggestions for everyday living. Includes community and CNIB resources. $12.50, Canadian funds

Low Vision: What You Can Do To Preserve - and Even Enhance - Your Usable Sight
by Helen Neal
Simon and Schuster, New York

A description of the programs, optical aids, and techniques that are a part of low vision services. Although this book is out of print, it is available in many public libraries.

Making Life More Livable
by Irving R. Dickman
American Foundation for the Blind (AFB)
15 West 16th Street
New York, NY 10011
(800) 232-5463   (212) 620-2000   FAX (212) 727-7418

Offers simple adaptations to make the home safer for people with vision impairment. $12.95 plus $3.00 shipping and handling. Also available on four-track audiocassette from regional branches of the National Library Service for the Blind and Physically Handicapped. RC 22319.

One Way or Another: A Guide to Independence for the Visually Impaired and Their Families
by Vivian Younger and Jill Sardegna
Sardegna Productions
710 Almondwood Way
San Jose, CA 95120
(408) 997-2150

Written by a vocational counselor who is visually impaired and a writer on disability issues, this book provides practical information for individuals and their families about living independently with vision loss. $15.00 plus $3.00 shipping and handling.

A Street to Share
Foundation Centre Louis-Hebert
525 boulevard Hamel Est, aile J
Quebec, Quebec G1M 2S8 Canada
(418) 529-6991

Presents typical situations experienced by individuals who are visually impaired or blind as they travel in their community. Makes suggestions for efficient and effective assistance. Videotape; U.S., $25.00

<u>Us and Them</u>
Fanlight Productions
47 Halifax St.
Boston, MA 02130
(617) 524-0980

Videotape about relationships between people who have disabilities and those who do not, including the relationship between a blind husband and a sighted wife. 32 minutes, black and white. Regular purchase price, $275.00; rental for one day $50.00; for one week $100.00; plus $9.00 shipping charge; call for possible discount.

Chapter 3

STARTING A SELF-HELP GROUP

It is estimated that there are approximately one half million self-help groups serving some 10 million people in the United States (U.S. Department of Health and Human Services: 1987). Both rehabilitation professionals and consumers agree that self-help groups make a unique contribution to the rehabilitation process for people who have experienced disabilities, including vision loss.

Self-help groups offer many benefits to participants, including learning how to deal with problems and needs; developing coping strategies; acquiring a feeling of empowerment or control over their lives; and combating isolation and alienation. Individuals who have experienced an increased feeling of isolation as a result of vision loss learn that others have experienced similar feelings. The feeling of isolation is common to individuals who have experienced disabilities, no matter what their educational or social background or their family situation. Self-help group members have often commented that their peers are more under-standing and patient than professional counselors, health care providers, or even family members, because they have had similar experiences. In addition, participants in self-help groups often hear about others' experiences with rehabilitation services; this information helps them to make the decision whether or not to enter into rehabilitation.

When the physician diagnoses progressive vision loss, even in the early stages, resources such as self-help groups should be mentioned. Patients may not absorb all of the physician's words, but if they are repeated at each visit, they will be remembered. A note in the patient's record serves to remind the physician to reinforce the suggestion on subsequent visits. Physicians, other health care providers, and rehabilitation professionals should avoid making the decision about self-help group participation for patients or clients. Individuals with vision loss themselves are the only ones capable of making the decision that they are ready to attend a self-help group.

When patients ask, "Do you have other patients with this condition?" it is time to make a referral to a self-help group. On return visits, service providers should ask patients or clients if they have attended the group. Their feedback will help professionals know whether the groups are providing the services the patients or clients need.

Rehabilitation Resource Manual: VISION Lexington, MA: Resources for Rehabilitation copyright 1993

Health care and rehabilitation professionals are ideally suited to identify and bring together individuals with common problems. However, professional service providers must understand that their role in initiating a self-help group is limited to helping to find participants; providing an initial site; and perhaps giving a presentation on medical aspects of eye diseases or rehabilitation services available in the community (Madara: undated).

If a professional is the catalyst for the formation of a group, he or she must disengage from this initial role to allow the group to develop autonomously. Since it is not unusual for professionals to encourage dependent client relationships, they must guard against this type of relationship if a group is to offer true mutual support.

A sense of group autonomy and "ownership" on the part of the members is essential to the success of the group. Members will invest their time and effort to make the group work as long as this sense of ownership lasts. If, however, group members sense that the group is "owned" by someone else, such as a health care professional or an agency, they often sit back and leave the work to the professionals.

Identifying a group facilitator or coordinator is the first step in developing a self-help group for people with vision loss. Weisse (1989) suggests identifying someone who has had group experience, in a vision loss support group, if possible. Former patients or clients who have had experience in coping with vision loss may be asked to start a group. Another method, especially useful in rural areas where no groups or services are available, is to identify an organized, articulate person who has experienced vision loss and has some background in a club or other organization. Announcements made in publications read by visually impaired individuals, at educational meetings, and posters on hospital and agency bulletin boards are also good recruitment techniques.

WHERE TO FIND EXISTING SELF-HELP GROUPS

In areas where self-help groups for people with vision loss are available, professionals can encourage self-referrals by providing a LARGE PRINT list of area groups along with their telephone numbers. The Community Services section found in the front of local telephone directories may list self-help groups for people with vision loss under "Health and Human Services" or "Disabilities." The "Social Service Organizations" section of the Yellow Pages is also a good source for locating the names of specific service agencies and information clearinghouses.

Public libraries often have local service directories. The reference librarian is available to help individuals find organizations which meet their needs. Hospital social services departments should know about the self-help groups in the area. The Information and Referral Service of the local United Way is another good source.

Staff at local agencies that serve individuals who are visually impaired or blind may also know where to find self-help groups. Self-help groups for people with other types of disabilities may be able to direct individuals to groups specifically for people with vision loss. Or they may welcome people with vision loss into their own disability group, especially when vision loss is secondary to another disabling condition such as multiple sclerosis, diabetes, or stroke.

Several national self-help clearinghouses are listed at the end of this chapter. These self-help clearinghouses are good resources for referrals to local self-help groups, literature, peer counseling training programs, and other appropriate resources.

When individuals are homebound, isolated due to lack of transportation, or where there are no support groups, alternative self-help networks offer benefits similar to those achieved by attending group meetings. Alternative self-help groups include telephone buddy systems and computer bulletin boards (Madara: 1992). For example, organizations that serve individuals who are visually impaired or blind may match individuals with similar diagnoses in order that they share practical information and provide emotional support through telephone conversations. Individuals participating in a telephone buddy network would be required to give permission to release their names and telephone numbers. Assistive technology such as LARGE PRINT or speech output enables individuals who are visually impaired or blind to access computer bulletin boards and share their experiences with others in similar situations, no matter what their location.

References

Madara, Edward J.
1992 "The Primary Value of a Self-Help Clearinghouse" pp. 117-124 in Alfred H. Katz et.al. Self-Help: Concepts and Applications Philadelphia, PA: The Charles Press, Publishers Developing Self-Help Groups - General Steps and Guidelines for Professionals Denville, NJ: New Jersey Self-Help Clearinghouse

U.S. Department of Health and Human Services
1987 The Surgeon General's Workshop on Self-Help and Public Health

Weisse, Fran A.
1989 "Self-Help Groups for People with Vision Loss" pp. 84-99 in Susan L. Greenblatt (ed.) Providing Services for People with Vision Loss: A Multidisciplinary Perspective Lexington, MA: Resources for Rehabilitation

PROFESSIONAL ORGANIZATIONS

Center for Self-Help Research
1918 University Avenue, Suite 3D
Berkeley, CA 94704
(415) 849-0731   FAX (415) 849-3402

Conducts research on self-help and disseminates results through publications.

National Self-Help Clearinghouse
Graduate School and University Center/CUNY
25 West 43rd Street
New York, NY 10036
(212) 642-2944

Conducts research; trains professionals to work with self-help groups. Maintains a national list of self-help clearinghouses and groups. Publications include "How to Organize a Self-Help Group," $6.00, "New Dimensions in Self-Help," $5.00, and a quarterly newsletter, "Self-Help Reporter," $10.00. A list of local self-help clearinghouses in the United States is available FREE by sending a self-addressed, stamped envelope.

PROFESSIONAL PUBLICATIONS

Amaral, Phyllis and LaDonna Ringering
1985 Peer Volunteers in Service Delivery to the Visually Impaired Santa Monica, CA: Center for the Partially Sighted

Arkansas Rehabilitation Research and Training Center
1981 Peer Counseling as a Rehabilitation Resource Author Hot Springs, AR: Arkansas Research and Training Center in Vocational Rehabilitation

Borkman, Thomasina (ed.)
1991 "Special Issue: Self-Help Research" American Journal of Community Psychology 19 (October)5

Byers-Lang, Rosalind E.
1984 "Peer Counselors, Network Builders for Elderly Persons" Journal of Visual Impairment and Blindness 78 (May) 5:193-197

De Balcazar, Yolanda Suarez, Tom Seekins, Adrienne Paine, Stephen B. Fawcett, and R. Mark Mathews
1989 "Self-Help and Social Support Groups for People with Disabilities: A Descriptive Report" in Rehabilitation Counseling Bulletin 33 (December) 2:151-158

Gimblett, Roberta
1992 Peer Mentoring: A Support Group Model for College Students with Disabilities Association on Higher Education and Disability, PO Box 21192, Columbus, OH 43221-0192

Haber, David
Professional Involvement in Self-Help Groups Omaha, NE: Creighton University's Center for Healthy Aging

Hill, Karen
1987 Helping You Helps Me: A Guide Book for Self-Help Groups Ottawa, Canada: Canadian Council on Social Development

Jacobs, Pearl L.
1984 "The Older Visually Impaired Person: A Vital Link in the Family and Community" Journal of Visual Impairment and Blindness 78 (April)4:154-162

Katz, Alfred H. and Eugene I. Bender
1990 Helping One Another: Self Help Groups in a Changing World Oakland, CA: Third Party Publishing Company
1976 The Strength In Us - Self-Help Groups in the Modern World New York, NY: New Viewpoints

Katz, Alfred H., Hannah L. Hedrick, Daryl Holtz Isenberg, Leslie M. Thompson, Therese Goodrich, and Austin H. Kutscher (eds.)
1992 Self-Help: Concepts and Applications Philadelphia, PA: The Charles Press, Publishers

Mallory, Lucretia
1984 Leading Self-Help Groups New York, NY: Family Service America

Rice, B. Douglas and Roy C. Farley
1987 Program Development and Management of Peer Counseling Services Hot Springs, AR: Arkansas Research and Training Center in Vocational Rehabilitation

Silverman, Phyllis R.
1986 "Foreword" in Support Networks in Massachusetts: A Listing of Self-Help Groups Massachusetts Cooperative Extension, Division of Home Economics, 113 Skinner Hall, University of Massachusetts, Amherst, MA 01003

Weisse, Fran A.

1989 "Self-Help Groups for People with Vision Loss" pp. 84-99 in Susan L. Greenblatt (ed.),
<u>Providing Services for People with Vision Loss: A Multidisciplinary Perspective</u>
Lexington, MA: Resources for Rehabilitation

REFERRAL RESOURCES

Organizations

(In the listings below, telephone numbers have symbols V for voice and TT for text telephone where organizations have published this information.)

The following national clearinghouses and self-help organizations can refer individuals to a self-help group in their area.

Association for Macular Diseases
210 East 64th Street
New York, NY 10021
(212) 605-3719

Membership organization which holds meetings in New York City area; helps to start chapters in other geographical areas; and arranges special programs in other parts of the country. Provides public education, support, and hot-line for people with macular degeneration. Membership, $20.00, includes newsletter.

Canadian Council on Social Concern
Self-Help Unit
PO Box 3505, 55 Parkdale Avenue
Ottawa, Ontario K1Y 4G1 Canada
(613) 728-1865

Develops policy on self-help issues, including those related to health. Newsletter, "Initiative: The Self-Help Newsletter," published in English and French, FREE.

CEF Crisis/Helpline, Inc.
36 Brinkerhoff Street
Plattsburgh, NY 12901
(518) 561-2330

Provides information and resources to self-help groups and advocates. Newsletter,"National Self-Help Network News." FREE

Lighthouse National Center for Vision and Aging (NCVA)
800 Second Avenue
New York, NY 10017
(800) 334-5497 (V/TT)   (212) 808-0077   FAX (212) 808-0110

Makes referrals to local support groups throughout the U.S. for adults who are visually impaired or blind.

National Self-Help Clearinghouse
Graduate School and University Center/CUNY
25 West 43rd Street, Room 620
New York, NY 10036
(212) 642-2944

Makes referral to local self-help groups. Publications include "How to Organize a Self-Help Group," $6.00, "New Dimensions in Self-Help," $5.00, and a quarterly newsletter, "Self-Help Reporter," $10.00. A list of local self-help clearinghouses in the U. S. is available by sending a self-addressed, stamped envelope. FREE

National Stargardt Self-Help Network
PO Box 136
West Chicago, IL 60186
(708) 208-5017

Network for individuals with Stargardt disease, a form of macular degeneration that usually appears before age 20. Includes families and individuals with allied macular dystrophies.

New Jersey Self-Help Clearinghouse
St. Clares Riverside Medical Center
25 Pocono Road
Denville, NJ 07834
(201) 625-7101   (201) 625-9053 (TT)   In NJ, (800) 367-6274

Makes referrals to local self-help groups. Publishes fact sheets such as "Ideas and Considerations for Starting a Self-Help Mutual Aid Group," "Suggestions on Locating a Meeting Place" and "Suggested Techniques for Recruiting Group Members." FREE

RP Foundation Fighting Blindness
1401 Mt. Royal Avenue
Baltimore, MD 21217
(800) 683-5555   (410) 225-9400   (410) 225-9409 (TT)
FAX (410) 225-3936

Local chapters, support groups, and information centers for people with retinitis pigmentosa. Refers individuals with Usher Syndrome to the Usher Syndrome Self-Help Network.

VISION Foundation, Inc.
818 Mt. Auburn Street
Watertown, MA 02172
(617) 926-4232   In MA, (800) 852-3029

Makes referrals to local self-help groups for individuals with vision loss.

Developing and Maintaining A Successful RP Support Group: A Directory of Ideas, Articles and Resources
RP Foundation Fighting Blindness
1401 Mt. Royal Avenue
Baltimore, MD 21217
(800) 683-5555   (410) 225-9400   (410) 225-9409 (TT)
FAX (410) 225-3936

Practical ideas for self-help groups. LARGE PRINT. FREE

Diabetes, Visual Impairment, and Group Support: A Guidebook
by Judith Caditz
The Center for the Partially Sighted
720 Wilshire Boulevard, Suite 200
Santa Monica, CA 90401-1713
(213) 458-3501

This guidebook is designed for individuals with diabetes and vision loss, their families, and the professionals who work with them. Offers suggestions for organizing education/support groups. Standard print and LARGE PRINT, $10.95 plus $2.50 shipping and handling.

Organizing Self-Help Groups: A Resource Guide
National Center for Education in Maternal and Child Health
2000 North 15th Street, Suite 701
Arlington, VA 22201
(703) 524-7802   FAX (703) 524-9335

Provides an annotated list of resources for organizing self-help groups and a list of self-help clearinghouses. FREE

Peer Counseling: A Small Group Approach
Arkansas Research and Training Center in Vocational Rehabilitation
PO Box 1358
Hot Springs, AR 71902
(501) 624-4411   FAX (501) 624-3515

Offers guidance to novice peer counselors in problem solving, assertiveness, and mutual support. Training package includes a trainer's manual, $6.00; participant's manual, $6.00; and a companion audiocassette, $5.00.

People Helping People: A Practical Guide for Mutual Support Groups
Frances J. Dory and Carol Eisman (eds.)
The Charles Press, PO Box 15715
Philadelphia, PA 19103
(215) 925-3995

Provides suggestions for new and established self-help groups. Includes catalogue of audio-visual materials, services, and national self-help organizations. $15.95

Plain Talk About Mutual Help Groups
c/o Consumer Information Center-2B
PO Box 100
Pueblo, CO 81002
(719) 948-3334

Provides an overview of mutual help groups and describes the benefits of sharing with others who have similar problems. FREE plus $1.00 service fee.

Resources for Self-Help Support Groups
VISION Foundation, Inc.
818 Mt. Auburn Street
Watertown, MA 02172
(617) 926-4232   In MA, (800) 852-3029

Lists literature, self-help clearinghouses, and offers suggestions for individuals with vision loss interested in setting-up self-help groups. LARGE PRINT. $5.00.

Self-Help/Mutual Aid Support Groups for Visually Impaired Older Persons: A Guide and Directory
Lighthouse National Center for Vision and Aging (NCVA)
800 Second Avenue
New York, NY 10017
(800) 334-5497 (V/TT)   (212) 808-0077   FAX (212) 808-0110

Lists local support groups throughout the U.S. $10.00

The Self-Help Sourcebook, fourth edition
American Self-Help Clearinghouse
Attn: Sourcebook
St. Clares Riverside Medical Center
Denville, NJ 07834
(201) 625-7101   (201) 625-9053 (TT)   In NJ, (800) 367-6274

Lists self-help groups throughout the U.S. $9.00; $10.00, first-class mail.

Chapter 4

SOURCES OF INFORMATION BY EYE DISEASE/CONDITION

MAJOR CAUSES OF VISION LOSS

CATARACTS

A cataract is a cloudiness or opacity in the lens of the eye which occurs most frequently in people over age 60. A common early symptom of cataracts is blurred vision, which may affect reading and night driving. Other symptoms include failing color perception and problems with glare and contrast. Sometimes cataracts are caused by eye inflammations, eye medications, or injury to the eye. The growth of a cataract is usually gradual and painless and may occur in one eye only or in both eyes at different rates.

Cataract surgery is one of the most common surgical procedures performed in the U.S. and has a high success rate. In some cases concurrent eye conditions prohibit cataract surgery or result in less than normal vision. A recent study (Sommer et al.: 1991) found a high rate of unoperated senile cataracts among blacks of all ages as well as among whites age 80 or older.

Prior to cataract surgery, the ophthalmologist and patient should discuss functional aspects affected by reduced vision due to cataract (such as driving, walking, and other activities), occupation, and general health as some of the determining factors for surgery. The patient's general physician and ophthalmologist should discuss the patient's other health problems and use of medications in order to determine the appropriate setting of the surgery, the type of anesthesia, and postoperative care.

Cataract surgery involves removal of the cataract; a substitute lens is provided by an intraocular lens implant, a contact lens, or cataract glasses, with intraocular lenses providing the best replication of normal vision (American Academy of Ophthalmology: 1988). Intraocular lenses also have the advantage of not requiring any special care after the surgery. Many individuals complain about glare after cataract surgery; this problem is often solved through the use of sunglasses. When reading, a black card with a window cut out is helpful in reducing the glare reflected from a page.

The National Eye Institute has funded the Age-Related Eye Disease Study, which is investigating the prevalence rates of cataract and macular degeneration and the effect of antioxidants and zinc in the role of cataract formation (National Eye Institute: 1990).

Most congenital cataracts are transmitted as a dominant trait, but recessive and sex-linked transmission have also been reported (Faye:1984). Congenital cataracts are much more difficult to treat surgically than cataracts in older adults. Acuity level and ability to tolerate glare are the major functional implications of congenital cataract. Some children may benefit from the use of low vision aids, such as reading lenses, telescopic devices, or absorptive lenses (sunglasses). If congenital cataracts are removed, contact lenses will be used. Individuals with congenital cataract should be advised to seek genetic counseling.

Children with cataracts should be referred for early intervention and special education programs (See Chapter 5, "Special Population Groups," Children and Adolescents). The ophthalmologist should be a member of the multidisciplinary team that meets with parents to develop an Individualized Education Plan (IEP). Reports on the child's visual condition should be provided to school personnel on a regular basis.

When vision is less than normal after cataract surgery in adults, the ophthalmologist should make a referral for rehabilitation services such as Talking Books, orientation and mobility instruction, and rehabilitation teaching.

References

American Academy of Ophthalmology
1988 "Cataract Surgery in the 1980's" Ophthalmology Instrument and Book Supplement
    54-64

Faye, Eleanor E.
1984 "Case Management in Twenty-six Common Conditions" Clinical Low Vision Boston,
    MA: Little, Brown and Company

National Eye Institute
1990 Clinical Trials Supported by the National Eye Institute Bethesda, MD: NIH Publication
    No. 90-2910

Sommer, Alfred, James M. Tielsch, Joanne Katz, Harry A. Quigley, John D. Gottsch,
Jonathan C. Javitt, James F. Martone, Richard M. Royall, Kathe Witt, and Sandi Ezrine
1991 "Racial Differences in the Cause-Specific Prevalence of Blindness in East Baltimore New
    England Journal of Medicine 325(November 14):1412-7

Publications and Tapes

Cataracts
National Eye Institute
Building 31, Room 6A32
Bethesda, MD 20892
(301) 496-5248

Discusses causes, treatment, and research. Available in standard print (FREE) from NEI; LARGE PRINT (FREE) or audiocassette ($2.00) from VISION Foundation, Inc., 818 Mt. Auburn Street, Watertown, MA 02172

The Physician's Guide to Cataracts, Glaucoma and Other Eye Problems
by John Eden, M.D. and the Editors of Consumer Reports Books
Consumer Reports Books, Yonkers, NY

Written by an ophthalmologist for patients, this book discusses examinations and medical procedures. $18.95

Individuals with diabetes must receive routine ophthalmological examinations to detect diabetic eye disease. Most individuals with diabetes show some retinal abnormalities; about 60% develop retinopathy (Eye Research Institute: 1990). Both macular edema, a build-up of fluid in the macula, and proliferative retinopathy, where abnormal blood vessels develop on the surface of the retina, are causes of vision loss in people with diabetes. The National Eye Institute has funded clinical studies that concluded that laser photocoagulation for macular edema was effective in reducing vision loss and that photocoagulation should be considered in severe cases of proliferative retinopathy (National Eye Institute: 1990).

The primary care physician or diabetologist and the ophthalmologist should work together to provide optimal care. Although some highly trained diabetologists examine the retinas for indications of retinal pathologies, it is wise to inform patients that they should have regular examinations performed by ophthalmologists. A recent study indicated that improved screening for retinopathy in patients with Type I diabetes mellitus will not only save many person-years of eyesight but will also save society a substantial amount of money by decreasing the costs of government health care and economic subsidy programs (Javitt et al.: 1991).

Diabetes educators, who may be nurses, dieticians, physicians, or psychologists, teach people with diabetes how to manage their diabetes effectively (Cypress et al.: 1992). Certified by the American Association of Diabetes Educators, these service providers help patients to adjust their insulin to proper levels, teach glucose monitoring, and perform a variety of other educational services. Diabetes educators and physicians must work together to care for individuals with diabetes. It is also important that they make necessary referrals for rehabilitation services.

A comparison of individuals with low vision with individuals who are legally blind led Wing (1986) to conclude that "individuals with advanced diabetic retinopathy must first be given assistance while they are losing vision, not after they are legally blind." After the referral is made, rehabilitation professionals will find it helpful to consult with diabetologists, ophthalmologists, and diabetes educators. They must also take into account the other health problems caused by diabetes that may affect rehabilitation; these include neuropathy, heart problems, kidney disease, and general fatigue. Exercise, a common prescription for people with diabetes, may induce low blood sugar levels and therefore must be carefully monitored (Bernbaum et al.: 1989). Other physical problems caused by diabetes, such as neuropathy and fatigue, require that rehabilitation training and orientation and mobility lessons be planned to accommodate the individual's capacities. (Bernbaum: 1991)

The fluctuation in vision that occurs with diabetic retinopathy is very stressful and affects the individual's ability to follow directions given by professionals and to cope with everyday life. Individual counseling from mental health professionals; support groups led by professional social workers; diabetes education programs; and self-help groups may help individuals with diabetes and vision loss cope with their emotions and the physical problems associated with diabetes. As with all conditions that cause progressive vision loss, it is wise to refer individuals for rehabilitation at an early stage; this enables them to prepare themselves psychologically and to learn about the various services and devices that can help them cope successfully with their vision loss.

To manage their diabetes, many people use a wide range of adapted equipment such as scales and thermometers with speech output, syringe magnifiers, and adapted insulin gauges. Several companies have added speech output devices to their blood glucose monitors. Diabetes educators, physicians, pharmacists, and sales representatives provide training in the proper use of these instruments. The Diabetics Division of the National Federation of the Blind, listed below, publishes a list of manufacturers of special equipment.

References

Bernbaum, Marla
1991 "Diabetes and Vision Loss" pp. 49-60 in Susan L. Greenblatt (ed.), Meeting the Needs of People with Vision Loss: A Multidisciplinary Perspective Lexington, MA: Resources for Rehabilitation

Bernbaum, Marla, Stewart G. Albert, and Jerome D. Cohen
1989 "Exercise Training in Individuals with Diabetic Retinopathy and Blindness" Archives of Physical Medicine and Rehabilitation 70(August):605-611

Cypress, Marjore, Judith Wylie-Rosett, Samuel S. Engel, and Terry B. Stager
1992 "The Scope of Practice of Diabetes Educators in a Metropolitan Area" The Diabetes Educator 18(Mar/Apr)2:111-114

Eye Research Institute
1990 "Diabetes and Your Eyes" Sundial Boston, MA: Eye Research Institute

Javitt, Jonathan C., Lloyd Paul Aiello, Lauri J. Bassi, Yen P. Chiang, and Joseph K. Canner
1991 "Detecting and Treating Retinopathy in Patients with Type I Diabetes Mellitus" Ophthalmology 98(October):1565-74

National Eye Institute
1990 Clinical Trials Supported by the National Eye Institute Bethesda, MD: NIH Publication No. 90-2910

Wing, Rena R.
1986 "Diabetes and Vision Loss: Improving the Services of the American Diabetes Association" Diabetes Care 9:95-6.

American Association of Diabetes Educators (AADE)
444 North Michigan Avenue, Suite 1240
Chicago, IL 60611
(800) 338-3633   (312) 644-2233

Membership organization for health care professionals who work with people with diabetes. Holds annual meeting. Publishes a bimonthly journal, "The Diabetes Educator," $45.00.

American Diabetes Association (ADA)
1660 Duke Street
Alexandria, VA 22314
(800) 232-3472   In Washington, DC area, (703) 549-1500
FAX (703) 836-7439

Membership in professional section is open to all professionals involved in the care of people with diabetes. Holds symposia; publishes journals, including "Diabetes," "Diabetes Care," and "Diabetes Spectrum."

National Diabetes Information Clearinghouse (NDIC)
Box NDIC
9000 Rockville Pike
Bethesda, MD 20892
(301) 468-2162

Clearinghouse for information on all aspects of diabetes. Publishes public and professional education materials and specialized bibliographies. Publications list, FREE.

National Eye Health Education Program
PO Box 20/20
Bethesda, MD 20892
(800) 869-2020   (301) 496-5248

Provides the "Educating People with Diabetes Kit," which includes an educator's guide, brochures, posters, fact sheets, and a press release. FREE

Bernbaum, Marla, Steward G. Albert, Stephanie R. Brusca, Ami Drimmer, Paul N. Duckro, Jerome D. Cohen, Mario C. Trindade, and Alan B. Silverberg
1989 "A Model Clinical Program for Patients with Diabetes and Vision Impairment" The Diabetes Educator 15:4:325-9

Cleary, Margaret E. and Christopher Fahy
1989 "Lighting a Lamp for Persons Who Are Visually Challenged" The Diabetes Educator 15:4:331-5.

Davidson, Mayer B.
1991 Diabetes Mellitus: Diagnosis and Treatment Third Edition New York, NY: Churchill Livingston

Dyer, Nancy and Pat Homeyer
1979 A Practical Education Program for the Diabetic Client Within the Rehabilitation Setting New York, NY: American Foundation for the Blind

Gambert, Steven R. (ed.)
1990 Diabetes Mellitus in the Elderly New York, NY: Raven Press

Herman, W., M. Halpern, B.E. Pack, J. Beasley, and C. Callaghan
1985 "Improving Eye Care for Persons with Diabetes Mellitus" JAMA 254:23:3293-4

Klein, R., E.L. Barrett-Connor, B.A. Blunt, and D.L. Wingard
1991 "Visual Impairment and Retinopathy in People with Normal Glucose Tolerance, Impaired Glucose Tolerance, and Newly Diagnosed NIDDM" Diabetes Care 14(10):914-18

Moss, Scot E., Ronald Klein, and Barbara E. K. Klein
1988 "The Incidence of Vision Loss in a Diabetic Population" Ophthalmology 95:10:1340-8

Nilsson, U.L.
1986 "Visual Rehabilitation of Patients with Advanced Diabetic Retinopathy" Documenta Ophthalmologica 62: 369-382

Oehler, Judith
1978 "Meeting the Psychosocial and Rehabilitative Needs of the Visually Impaired Diabetic" Journal of Visual Impairment and Blindness 72:358-361

Petzinger, Ruth A.
1992 "Diabetes Aids and Products for People with Visual or Physical Impairments" The Diabetes Educator 18(Mar/Apr)2:121-138

Stepien, Cathy J., Marilyn Bowbeer, and Roland G. Hiss
1992 "Screening for Diabetic Retinopathy in Communities" The Diabetes Educator
    18(Mar/Apr)2:115-120

Wulsin, Lawson R., Alan M. Jacobson, and Lawrence I. Rand
1987 "Psychosocial Aspects of Diabetic Retinopathy" Diabetes Care 10(May-June): 367-373

Zakov, Z.N.
1990 "Managing Diabetic Retinopathy" Cleveland Clinic Journal of Medicine 57(7):609-12

REFERRAL RESOURCES

Organizations

(In the listings below, telephone numbers have symbols V for voice and TT for text telephone where organizations have published this information.)

American Diabetes Association (ADA)
1660 Duke Street
Alexandria, VA 22314
(800) 232-3472   In Washington, DC area, (703) 549-1500
FAX (703) 836-7439

National office refers callers to local affiliate for education materials.   Membership, $24.00; includes discount on publications and quarterly newsletter, "Diabetes."

Canadian Diabetes Association (CDA)
78 Bond Street
Toronto, Ontario M5B 2J8 Canada
(416) 362-4440   FAX (416) 362-6849

Provides service and education to individuals with diabetes and supports research. Produces a variety of inexpensive educational brochures in English and French.

Diabetics Division
National Federation of the Blind (NFB)
811 Cherry Street, Suite 309
Columbia, MO 65201
(314) 875-8911

A national support and information network. Publishes a quarterly magazine, "Voice of the Diabetic," which includes personal experiences, medical information, recipes, and resources. Available in standard print and four-track audiocassette.   FREE sample.   Individual membership of $5.00 includes subscription. Nonmember subscription, $15.00. Also available, "Resource List: Aids and Appliances," a list of adaptive equipment; standard print and audiocassette, $1.00; braille, $2.00.

Juvenile Diabetes Foundation (JDF)
432 Park Avenue South
New York, NY 10016-8013
(800) 533-2873   (212) 889-7575   FAX (212) 725-7259

JDF in Canada:
4632 Yonge Street, Suite 100
Willowdale, Ontario M2N 5M1 Canada
(416) 223-1068

Raises funds to find the cause, cure, prevention, and treatment of diabetes and its complications. Local chapters provide parent-to-parent counseling and self-help groups for newly diagnosed diabetics and their families. FREE pamphlets and fact sheets. Membership, $25.00, includes subscription to magazine "Countdown."

National Diabetes Information Clearinghouse (NDIC)
Box NDIC
Bethesda, MD 20892
(301) 468-2162

National clearinghouse for information on all aspects of diabetes. Publishes public and professional education materials and specialized bibliographies. FREE list of publications.

Publications and Tapes

Diabetes and Your Eyes
"Sundial," Winter 1990
Schepens Eye Research Institute
20 Staniford Street
Boston, MA 02114
(617) 742-3140

Discusses causes, treatment, and research on visual complications by diabetes. FREE. Also available on audiocassette from VISION Foundation, Inc., 818 Mt. Auburn Street, Watertown, MA 02172, $2.00.

Diabetes: Caring For Your Emotions As Well As Your Health
by Jerry Edelwich and Archie Brodsky
Addison Wesley Publishing Company, Reading, MA

Although not specifically written for people with vision loss, this book offers suggestions for adaptations, relationships with medical personnel, family strategies, employment questions, technology, and support groups. $12.45

Diabetes Self-Management
PO Box 52890
Boulder, CO 80322-2890

A bimonthly magazine designed to help people with diabetes manage their conditions independently. Includes articles about special aids, diet, and diabetes education. U.S., $21.00; Canada, $24.00; foreign, $36.00.

Diabetes, Vision Loss and Aging
Lighthouse National Center for Vision and Aging (NCVA)
800 Second Avenue
New York, NY 10017
(800) 334-5497 (V/TT)   (212) 808-0077   FAX (212) 808-0110

A booklet with information about ocular complications of diabetes and management of medications for people with vision loss. Single copy, FREE; 2-99 copies, $.50 each

Diabetes, Visual Impairment, and Group Support: A Guidebook
by Judith Caditz
The Center for the Partially Sighted
720 Wilshire Boulevard, Suite 200
Santa Monica, CA 90401-1713
(213) 458-3501

Written by a woman with Type I diabetes, this guidebook is designed for individuals with diabetes and vision loss, their families, and professionals. Discusses diabetes mellitus, how it affects vision, psychosocial aspects, diet, adaptive aids, and organizing education/support groups. Standard print and LARGE PRINT, $10.95 plus $2.50 shipping and handling.

Diabetic Retinopathy
National Eye Institute (NEI)
Building 31, Room 6A32
Bethesda, MD 20892
(301) 496-5248

Discusses the effects of diabetes on the eyes; symptoms of diabetic retinopathy; treatment;

vitrectomy; and research. Available FREE in standard print from NEI; in LARGE PRINT (FREE) and audiocassette ($2.00) from VISION Foundation, Inc., 818 Mt. Auburn Street, Watertown, MA 02172.

Diabetic's Book: All Your Questions Answered
by June Bierman and Barbara Toohey
St Martin's Press, New York, NY

Discusses a wide variety of issues affecting people with diabetes, including diet, exercise, emotions, and other aspects of everyday living. $10.95

Don't Be Blind to Diabetes
Lions Clubs International, Public Relations Division
300 22nd Street
Oak Brook, IL 60521
(708) 571-5466   FAX (718) 571-8890

Discusses the early detection of diabetes, its effect on vision, and interviews with patients and experts in the field. 19 minutes. Videotape (VHS or Beta) $25.00; 16mm film $100.00

Exchange Lists for Meal Planning
American Diabetes Association (ADA)
1970 Chain Bridge Road
McLean, VA 22109-0592
(800) 232-3472   In Washington, DC area, (703) 549-1500

These exchange lists are available in LARGE PRINT, $2.50 plus $1.75 shipping and handling. Also available on four-track audiocassette (must be played on NLS audiocassette player) from the Diabetics Division, National Federation of the Blind, $2.00; braille, $15.00   (See "ORGANIZATIONS" section above.)

Know Your Diabetes, Know Yourself
Joslin Diabetes Center, Attention: Accounting Dept.
One Joslin Place
Boston, MA 02215
(617) 732-2429   FAX (617) 732-2664

Videotape in which Joslin patients (not actors) talk about the daily issues of diabetes management: using an eating plan; the important roles exercise, monitoring, injections, and foot and eye care play in their lives; and how they manage their disease when sick or traveling. Joslin health professionals discuss the essentials of good diabetes care. 60 minutes. $39.95 VHS format.

<u>Living with Diabetes</u> $2.00
<u>Living with Diabetic Retinopathy</u> $1.75
Resources for Rehabilitation
33 Bedford Street, Suite 19A
Lexington, MA 02173
(617) 862-6455   FAX (617) 861-7517

Designed for distribution by professionals, these LARGE PRINT (18 point bold type) publications describe the disease, service providers, and organizations, devices, and publications. Minimum purchase 25 copies per title. Discounts for orders of 100 or more copies. See order form on last page of book. See order form on last page of book.

<u>1992 Buyer's Guide To Diabetes Products</u>
American Diabetes Association (ADA)
1970 Chain Bridge Road
McLean, VA 22109-0592
(800) 232-3472   In Washington, DC area, (703) 549-1500

Compares products from a variety of manufacturers of syringes, insulin pumps, etc. $2.95 plus $1.75 shipping and handling

GLAUCOMA

Glaucoma is a group of eye diseases which cause increased pressure of the fluid in the eye; changes in the optic disk; and losses in the visual field. Glaucoma is far more prevalent among black Americans than among white Americans. A study of a random sample of Medicare recipients 65 years or older concluded that blacks do not receive surgery for glaucoma as frequently as whites (Javitt et al.: 1991)

Often the individual experiences no symptoms; only an ophthalmic examination will detect elevated intraocular pressure, damage to the optic disk, and in some cases, loss of peripheral vision that the patient has not noticed. Some individuals experience blurred vision, redness of the eye, or pain. When undiagnosed or left untreated, glaucoma can lead to blindness. Early diagnosis and treatment can prevent much vision loss from glaucoma. Experts recommend that everyone over the age of 35 have an eye examination with an intraocular pressure check every two years. The National Eye Institute has sponsored several studies that are investigating experimental treatments for glaucoma, including trabeculectomy, argon laser treatment, and fluorouracil filtering surgery (National Eye Institute: 1990).

Because glaucoma usually begins with a loss of peripheral vision, individuals may benefit from orientation and mobility training to help them travel safely. The state agency that serves individuals who are visually impaired or blind may provide these services or may refer individuals to a private agency or a private practitioner.

References

Javitt, Jonathan C., A. Marshall McBean, Geraldine A. Nicholson, J. Daniel Babish, Joan L. Warren, and Henry Krakauer
1991 "Undertreatment of Glaucoma Among Black Americans" New England Journal of Medicine 325(November 14):1418-22

National Eye Institute
1990 Clinical Trials Supported by the National Eye Institute Bethesda, MD: NIH Publication No. 90-2910

Foundation for Glaucoma Research
490 Post Street, Suite 1042
San Francisco, CA 94102
(415) 986-3162

Supports research into the causes and treatment of glaucoma through a fellowship program for ophthalmologists and the maintenance of a clinical database. Operates an eye donor network, which enables researchers to study the eyes donated by glaucoma patients and their families.

Glaucoma Foundation
310 East 14th Street
New York, NY 10003
(800) 832-3926   (212) 260-1000

Supports research into the causes and treatment of glaucoma.

National Eye Health Education Program
PO Box 20/20
Bethesda, MD 20892
(800) 869-2020   (301) 496-5248

Produces "Don't Lose Sight of Glaucoma," a community education kit that includes information on establishing a community outreach program, posters, fact sheets, and public service announcements. FREE

National Glaucoma Research
American Health Assistance Foundation
15825 Shady Grove Road, Suite 140
Rockville, MD 20850
(800) 437-2423   (301) 948-3244

Funds research into the causes of glaucoma and development of new treatments. Publishes public education booklets. Newsletter, "National Glaucoma Research Report," FREE.

REFERRAL RESOURCES

Organizations

<u>Foundation for Glaucoma Research</u>
490 Post Street, Suite 1042
San Francisco, CA 94102
(415) 986-3162

Offers public education program; telephone support network; quarterly newsletter, "Gleams," FREE. Operates an eye donor network, which enables researchers to study the eyes donated by glaucoma patients and their families.

<u>Glaucoma Foundation</u>
310 East 14th Street
New York, NY 10003
(800) 832-3926   (212) 260-1000   FAX (212) 260-1002

Operates a direct response hot-line. Publishes "About Glaucoma" and "Glaucoma Medications - Purpose and Side Effects." Single copies, FREE

<u>National Glaucoma Research</u>
American Health Assistance Foundation
15825 Shady Grove Road, Suite 140
Rockville, MD 20850
(800) 437-2423   (301) 948-3244

Toll-free hotline offers current information on research, treatments, and publications. Quarterly newsletter, "National Glaucoma Research Report," FREE.

<u>National Society to Prevent Blindness</u> (NSPB)
500 East Remington Road
Schaumburg, IL 60173-4557
(800) 221-3004   (708) 843-2020   FAX (708) 843-8458

NSPB sponsors glaucoma screenings through local chapters and produces public and professional materials on many eye conditions, including glaucoma. FREE catalogue.

Glaucoma
National Eye Institute (NEI)
NIH, Building 31, Room 6A32
Bethesda, MD 20892
(301) 496-5248

Brochure that describes open-angle glaucoma, treatment, and current research. Available FREE in standard print from NEI; in LARGE PRINT (FREE) and audiocassette ($2.00) from VISION Foundation, Inc., 818 Mt. Auburn Street, Watertown, MA 02172.

Glaucoma - Vision's Insidious Thief
"Sundial" Spring, 1988
Schepens Eye Research Institute
20 Staniford Street
Boston, MA 02114
(617) 742-3140

A report on glaucoma with a glossary, treatment options, medications, and research. Available in standard print from the Eye Research Institute (FREE) and audiocassette ($2.00) from VISION Foundation, 818 Mt. Auburn Street, Watertown, MA 02172.

The Physician's Guide to Cataracts, Glaucoma and Other Eye Problems
by John Eden, M.D. and the Editors of Consumer Reports Books
Consumer Reports Books, Yonkers, NY

Written by an ophthalmologist for patients, this book discusses examinations and medical procedures. $18.95

Some Answers About Glaucoma
American Health Assistance Foundation
15825 Shady Grove Road, Suite 140
Rockville, MD 20850
(800) 437-2423   In MD, (301) 948-3244

Describes the major types of glaucoma, risk factors, diagnosis and treatment, and lists helpful references, toll-free numbers, and organizations. LARGE PRINT. FREE

<u>Understanding and Living With Glaucoma: A Reference Guide For Patients and Their Families</u>
Foundation for Glaucoma Research
490 Post Street, Suite 1042
San Francisco, CA 94102
(415) 986-3162

Written by a person with glaucoma, this booklet describes living with a chronic health condition. Standard print, English and Spanish. Single copy FREE. English version audiocassette ($2.00) available from VISION Foundation, Inc., 818 Mt. Auburn Street, Watertown, MA 02172

MACULAR DEGENERATION

The most common form of age-related macular degeneration, the drusenoid or "dry" form, involves atrophy of the macula; there is no current treatment. The neovascular or "wet" form, in which serum and abnormal blood vessels develop, may sometimes be treated by laser, depending upon the location of the lesion and a variety of other factors. The Macular Photocoagulation Study, supported by the National Eye Institute, determined that laser treatment is effective, at least initially, in preventing severe visual loss from the neovascular type of macular disease (National Eye Institute: 1983); however, Bressler et al. report that "Even in successfully treated cases, severe visual loss is postponed only for about 18 months because of the high rate of recurrent CNVMs [choroidal neovascular membranes] that extend into the fovea" (1988:375).

Recently, several groups of ophthalmologists have attempted to remove subretinal neovascular membranes surgically, although the number of subjects who have had this procedure is small. To date, the results of this surgical excision are inconclusive, with some investigators reporting positive outcomes (Lambert et al.: 1992) and others finding that surgery does not result in positive outcomes for age-related macular degeneration (Berger and Kaplan: 1992; Thomas et al.: 1992; Vander et al.: 1991). Another type of therapy that has been suggested is a dietary supplement of vitamins that are known to be antioxidants; it is hypothesized that they prevent the development of neovascular membranes (see, for example, Gerster: 1991; Goldberg et al.: 1988). The National Eye Institute has funded the Age-Related Eye Disease Study, which is investigating the prevalence rates of macular degeneration and cataract as well as the effects of antioxidants and zinc on these conditions (National Eye Institute: 1990).

Data from the National Institute on Aging suggest an association between age-related macular degeneration and cataract (Liu et al: 1989) and that both may result from related processes, including exposure to light. The authors suggest that cataract removal may place the individual at greater risk for developing age-related macular degeneration and that lens implants which reduce the transmittance of ultraviolet light be used.

Best disease or vitelliform macular degeneration is a hereditary form of the macular degeneration passed on by dominant genes and is usually detected in a child's early years. Stargardt's disease, also known as fundus flavimaculatus or juvenile macular dystrophy, is passed on by recessive genes and is usually detected in the teen-age years.

Low vision aids are currently the only available treatment for the majority of individuals who have macular degeneration (Bressler et al: 1988). Ophthalmologists and optometrists should refer individuals to low vision services. Individuals with macular degeneration are often able to use low vision aids successfully. It is commonly thought that people who have macular degeneration do not have mobility problems, since the disease affects the central vision. However, some individuals do have problems with travel and would benefit from orientation and mobility training.

References

Berger, Adam S. and Henry J. Kaplan
1992 "Clinical Experience with the Surgical Removal of Subfoveal Neovascular Membranes" Ophthalmology 99(June):969-76

Bressler, Neil M., Susan B. Bressler, and Stuart L. Fine
1988 "Age-Related Macular Degeneration" Survey of Ophthalmology 32:6:375-413

Gerster, Helga
1991 "Review: Antioxidant Protection of the Ageing Macula" Age and Ageing 20:60-69

Goldberg, Jack, Gordon Flowerdew, Ellen Smith, Jacob A. Brody, and Mark O.M. Tso
1988 "Factors Associated with Age-Related Macular Degeneration" American Journal of Epidemiology 128:701-710

Lambert, H. Michael, Antonio Capone, Thomas M. Aaberg, Paul Sternberg, Barry A. Mandell, and Pedro F. Lopez
1992 "Surgical Excision of Subfoveal Neovascular Membranes in Age-Related Macular Degeneration" American Journal of Ophthalmology 113(March):257-62

Liu, Ingrid Y., Lois White, and Andrea LaCroix
1989 "The Association of Age-Related Macular Degeneration and Lens Opacities in the Aged" American Journal of Public Health 79:765-769

National Eye Institute
1990 Clinical Trials Supported by the National Eye Institute Bethesda, MD: NIH Publication No. 90-2910
1983 Vision Research: A National Plan Bethesda, MD

Thomas, Matthew A., Gilbert Grand, David F. Williams, Carol M. Lee, Samuel R. Pesin, and Marc A. Lowe
1992 "Surgical Management of Subfoveal Choroidal Neovascularization" Ophthalmology 99(June):952-968

Vander, James F., Jay L. Federman, Craig Greven, M. Madison Slusher, and Veit-Peter Gabel
1991 "Surgical Removal of Massive Subretinal Hemorrhage Associated with Age-related Macular Degeneration" Ophthalmology 98(January):23-27

PROFESSIONAL ORGANIZATIONS

Macular Disease Research Center
Schepens Eye Research Institute
20 Staniford Street
Boston, MA 02114
(617) 742-3140

Studies causes and symptoms of hereditary and age-related macular degeneration.

PROFESSIONAL PUBLICATIONS

Collee, Christine M., Alex E. Jalkh, John J. Weiter, and Gerald R. Friedman
1985 "Visual Improvement with Low Vision Aids in Stargardt's Disease" Ophthalmology
    92:1657-1659

Hampton, G. Robert and Philip T. Nelsen (eds.)
1992 Age-Related Macular Degeneration Principles and Practice New York, NY: Raven
    Press

Harris, Michael J., David Robins, Joseph M. Dieter, Stuart L. Fine, and David Guyton
1985 "Eccentric Visual Acuity in Patients with Macular Disease" Ophthalmology 92:1550-
    1553

Lovie-Kitchin, Jan E. and Kenneth J. Bowman
1985 Senile Macular Degeneration Stoneham, MA: Butterworth

Nilsson, U.L. and S.E. Nilsson
1986 "Rehabilitation of the Visually Handicapped with Advanced Macular Degeneration"
    Documenta Ophthalmologica 62: 345-367

Organizations

Association for Macular Diseases
210 East 64th Street
New York, NY 10021
(212) 605-3719

Membership organization which produces newsletter and holds meetings in New York and other areas. Provides public education, support, and hot-line for macular degeneration patients. Membership, $20.00

National Stargardt Self-Help Network
PO Box 136
West Chicago, IL 60186
(708) 208-5017

Support network for individuals with Stargardt disease, their families, and individuals with allied macular dystrophies.

Publications and Tapes

Age-Related Macular Degeneration
National Eye Institute (NEI)
Building 31, Room 6A32
Bethesda, MD 20892
(301) 496-5248

A brochure that discusses symptoms of age-related macular degeneration, treatment, and research. FREE in standard print from NEI; in LARGE PRINT (FREE) and audiocassette ($2.00) from VISION Foundation, Inc., 818 Mt. Auburn Street, Watertown, MA 02172

Coping with the Diagnosis of Sight Loss
Resources for Rehabilitation
33 Bedford Street, Suite 19A
Lexington, MA 02173
(617) 862-6455   FAX (617) 861-7517

An audiocassette in which three consumers, one of whom has macular degeneration, discuss their reactions and experiences when told that they were losing their vision. $12.00 plus $3.00 shipping and handling.

I Keep Five Pairs of Glasses in a Flower Pot
by Henrietta Levner
National Association for the Visually Handicapped (NAVH)
22 West 21st Street
New York, NY 10010
(212) 889-3141

Describes an older woman's experience learning to live with low vision due to macular degeneration. LARGE PRINT. $2.00

Living with Age-Related Macular Degeneration
Resources for Rehabilitation
33 Bedford Street, Suite 19A
Lexington, MA 02173
(617) 862-6455   FAX (617) 861-7517

Designed for distribution by professionals, this LARGE PRINT (18 point bold type) publication describes service organizations and publications that help people with macular degeneration. Minimum purchase, 25 copies. $1.25 per copy plus shipping and handling. Discounts available for purchases of 100 or more copies. See order form on last page of this book.

Look Out for Annie
Lighthouse National Center for Vision and Aging (NCVA)
800 Second Avenue
New York, NY 10017
(800) 334-5497 (V/TT)   (212) 808-0077   FAX (212) 808-0110

This videotape portrays an older woman with macular degeneration and her interactions with her family and friends. Discussion guide included. $25.00, VHS or BETA format.

Out of the Corner of My Eye: Living With Vision Loss in Later Life
by Nicolette Pernod Ringgold
American Foundation for the Blind (AFB)
15 West 16th Street
New York, NY 10011
(800) 232-5463   (212) 620-2000   FAX (212) 620-2105

Written by a woman who became legally blind in her late 70's due to macular degeneration, this book offers practical advice and encouragement for elders with vision loss. LARGE PRINT and audiocassette, $14.95 plus $3.00 shipping and handling.

RETINITIS PIGMENTOSA

Retinitis pigmentosa (RP) is an inherited eye disease which causes degeneration of the retina's photoreceptor cells. Night blindness and peripheral vision loss are symptoms of rod cell degeneration; decreased central vision and loss of color vision are symptoms of cone cell degeneration. Retinitis pigmentosa is difficult to diagnose, but as it progresses retinal changes may be detected by electroretinogram (ERG) and visual field and visual function tests. The progression of symptoms is unpredictable and varies with the genetic forms of the disease. No treatment for retinitis pigmentosa is available.

Usher syndrome is an inherited disorder which involves retinitis pigmentosa, hearing loss, and in some cases, balance problems. In individuals with Usher syndrome Type I, there is profound hearing loss at birth, retinitis pigmentosa, and balance problems. Individuals with Type II have moderate to severe hearing loss and retinitis pigmentosa but have no balance problems.

Service providers should be certain that individuals with retinitis pigmentosa receive genetic counseling in order to understand the hereditary patterns of their specific variant of this retinal condition, especially if the patients or their offspring are planning on having children.

Patients with retinitis pigmentosa should be referred for additional rehabilitation counseling and training as vision decreases. Determining when a referral is necessary may be difficult as individuals often are reluctant to admit, even to themselves, that their vision has deteriorated. Asking questions about specific tasks that the individual undertakes may be the best way to assess whether visual function has deteriorated to the point where additional help is necessary. Despite the fact that they have night blindness and tunnel vision, some individuals with retinitis pigmentosa resist using a white cane for safe mobility. Talking with peers in a self-help support group setting may enable them to accept both the cane and orientation and mobility training.

(In the listings below, telephone numbers have symbols V for voice and TT for text telephone where organizations have published this information.)

Alliance of Genetic Support Groups
35 Wisconsin Circle, Suite 440
Chevy Chase, MD 20815
(800) 336-4363   (301) 652-5553   FAX (301) 654-0171

A coalition of support groups for consumers and professionals concerned with genetic diseases. Sponsors national conferences and publishes monthly newsletter, "Alliance Alert." Membership, individuals, $15.00; groups, $40.00.

RP Foundation Fighting Blindness
1401 Mt. Royal Avenue
Baltimore, MD 21217
(800) 683-5555   (410) 225-9400   (410) 225-9409 (TT)
FAX (410) 225-3936

Provides research grants for scientists and ophthalmologists who study retinitis pigmentosa and other retinal degenerative diseases; maintains national registry and retina donor program.

PROFESSIONAL PUBLICATIONS

Fillman, R.D., L.E. Leguire, and M. Sheridan
1989 "Considerations for Serving Adolescents with Usher's Syndrome" RE:view 21 (1), 19-25

Pagon, Roberta A.
1988 "Retinitis Pigmentosa" Survey of Ophthalmology 33:3:137-77

Heckenlively, John R.
1988 Retinitis Pigmentosa Philadelphia, PA: J.B. Lippincott Co.

REFERRAL RESOURCES

Organizations

(In the listings below, telephone numbers have symbols V for voice and TT for text telephone where organizations have published this information.)

<u>RP Foundation Fighting Blindness</u>
1401 Mt. Royal Avenue
Baltimore, MD 21217
(800) 683-5555   (410) 225-9400   (410) 225-9409 (TT)
FAX (410) 225-3936

Supports research, retina donor program, and national RP registry. Provides public and professional education materials and quarterly newsletter, "Fighting Blindness News," available in LARGE PRINT, audiocassette, and braille. Local chapters, support groups, and information centers. Publishes "Information about RP and Allied Retinal Degenerative Diseases," "The RP Backgrounder," "Information About Usher Syndrome," and "Usher Syndrome Backgrounder." LARGE PRINT. FREE

<u>RP International</u>
PO Box 900
Woodland Hills, CA 91365
(800) 344-4877   (818) 992-0500

Information clearinghouse; public education materials. Provides counseling, referrals, and supports research. Newsletter, "The Night Lighter," available in LARGE PRINT.

<u>Texas Association of RP</u> (TARP)
PO Box 8388
Corpus Christi, TX 78468-8388
(512) 852-8515

Clearinghouse for RP information; quarterly newsletter, "RP Messenger," provides support and information for RP patients.

<u>Usher Syndrome Project/Genetics</u>
Boys Town National Research Hospital
555 North 30 Street
Omaha, NE 68131
(800) 835-1468 (V/TT)   In NE, (404) 498-6742

Conducts research to locate the gene(s) which cause Usher syndrome. Families are needed to participate in the research.

The Business of Living Publications
by Dorothy H. Stiefel
PO Box 8388
Corpus Christi, TX 78468-8388
(512) 852-3993

A series of booklets about dealing with retinitis pigmentosa and vision loss: "Dealing with the Threat of Loss" focuses on aspects of daily living with RP from diagnosis to coping. Bold-face type, $4.50; audiocassette: English, $6.00; Spanish or French, $7.50. Add postage and handling, U.S., $2.00; Canada, $3.00.

"Stress and Well-Being" offers ways to deal with the stress of everyday living which is intensified for an individual with inconsistent vision. Bold-face type: $4.50; audiocassette: English only, $6.00. Add postage and handling, U.S., $2.00; Canada, $3.00.

"The 'Madness' of Usher's: Coping with Vision and Hearing Loss" describes the author's experience in living with Type II Usher syndrome. Standard print, $7.50; audiocassette, $12.50. Add postage and handling, U.S., $2.00; Canada, $3.00.

Coping with the Diagnosis of Sight Loss
Resources for Rehabilitation
33 Bedford Street, Suite 19A
Lexington, MA 02173
(617) 862-6455   FAX (617) 861-7517

An audiocassette in which three consumers, one of whom has retinitis pigmentosa, discuss their reactions and experiences when told that they were losing their vision. $12.00 plus $3.00 shipping and handling.

The Inheritance of RP and Allied Retinal Degenerative Diseases
by Jill C. Hennessey
RP Foundation Fighting Blindness
1401 Mt. Royal Avenue
Baltimore, MD 21217
(800) 683-5555   (410) 225-9400   (410) 225-9409 (TT)
FAX (410) 225-3936

A booklet that describes the basic genetics and inheritance patterns of retinitis pigmentosa, including autosomal dominant, autosomal recessive, and x-linked (sex linked). Defines allied retinal degenerative diseases such as Best disease, Stargardt disease, choroideremia, and Usher syndrome. Glossary. Lists RP Research Centers. Available in LARGE PRINT, audio-cassette, and braille. FREE

Usher's Syndrome: What It Is, How to Cope, and How to Help
by Earlene Duncan, Hugh T. Prickett, Dan Finkelstein, McCay Vernon, and Toni Hollingsworth
Charles C. Thomas, Springfield, IL

Includes interviews with individuals with Usher syndrome, psychological adjustment to the diagnosis, and educational and vocational concerns. $24.75 plus $3.00 shipping and handling.

AIDS AND VISION LOSS

A number of pathological ocular conditions occur in patients with AIDS. The most common of these conditions, cotton wool spots, appear as lesions in the retina and do not usually cause decreased acuity. According to Heinemann (1992), it is important that cotton wool spots be properly diagnosed so that they are not confused with cytomegalovirus (CMV), an infection of the retina that can lead to severe visual impairment or blindness if untreated. The cause and prevalence of CMV are unknown, although it has been estimated that 20 to 25 percent of patients with AIDS develop this virus (National Eye Institute: 1990). Numerous observers have suggested that the prevalence rate will increase as treatment of patients with AIDS improves and their life spans are extended. The Food and Drug Administration has approved two drugs for the treatment of retinal CMV: ganciclovir and foscarnet. The side effects of these drugs may be serious; both drugs are administered intravenously and require an in-dwelling catheter for the daily treatments that must be continued for the rest of the patient's life in order to control the progression of the virus, although neither drug cures retinal CMV (Holland: 1992). A study sponsored by the National Institutes of Health concluded that patients who receive foscarnet survive four months longer than those who receive ganciclovir (NIH: 1991). The study directors concluded that foscarnet may be the drug of choice, except for patients who have decreased renal function.

Other effects of AIDS on vision include damage to the optic nerve, causing a decrease in contrast sensitivity and color discrimination (Quiceno et al.: 1992). Nonviral infections, parasitic diseases, and Kaposi's sarcoma, which affects the eyelids or conjunctiva, are also associated with AIDS.

Because of the serious side effects of ganciclovir and foscarnet, it is important that the primary care physician and the ophthalmologist work cooperatively to minimize side effects while attempting to preserve vision. The rehabilitation professional working with the patient should be informed of the patient's physical condition to determine his or her ability to participate in rehabilitation. Patients who are too weak to actively participate in rehabilitation may benefit from talking books, volunteer readers, radio reading services, or descriptive video services.

References

Heinemann, M.H.
1992 "Ophthalmic Problems" Medical Management of AIDS Patients, The Medical Clinics of North America 76(January)1:83-97

Holland, Gary N.
1992 "Acquired Immunodeficiency Syndrome and Ophthalmology: The First Decade" American Journal of Ophthalmology 114(July):86-94

National Eye Institute
1990 Clinical Trials Supported by the National Eye Institute Bethesda, MD NIH Publication No. 90-2910, p. 55

National Institutes of Health
1991 Clinical Alert to Physicians and Others who Treat Patients with AIDS October 17

Quinceno, Jose Ivan, Edmund Capparelli, Alfredo A. Sadun, David Munguia, Igor Grant, Alan Listhaus, Joseph Crapotta, Brent Lambert, and William R. Freeman
1992 "Visual Dysfunction without Retinitis in Patients with Acquired Immunodeficiency Syndrome" American Journal of Ophthalmology 113(January):8-13

PROFESSIONAL ORGANIZATIONS

(In the listings below, telephone numbers have symbols V for voice and TT for text telephone where organizations have published this information.)

National AIDS Information Clearinghouse (NAIC)
PO Box 6003
Rockville, MD 20850
(800) 458-5231   (800) 344-7012 (TT)   (800) 874-2572 (clinical trials)

Operated by the Centers for Disease Control, this is an information service for professionals who work with people with AIDS. Provides information about organizations that provide services to people with AIDS, funding sources, and clinical trials. Provides technical assistance to organizations and state health departments. Makes referrals to patient support groups and other service organizations that provide services to people with AIDS. Publishes a calendar of conferences that relate to AIDS.

National Institute of Allergy and Infectious Diseases (NIAID)
National Institutes of Health
Building 31, Room 7A32
Bethesda, MD 20892
(800) 874-2572 for information on clinical trials

Supports clinical and basic research related to AIDS and other infectious diseases. "NIAID AIDS Agenda" discusses new developments and the establishment of research centers and "NIAID Dateline" summarizes recent research and developments. FREE

AIDS Clinical Care, Massachusetts Medical Society, PO Box 9085, Waltham, MA 02254

AIDS/HIV Treatment Directory, AmFar, 733 Third Avenue, 12th Floor, New York, NY 10017

AIDS Targeted Information/ATIN, Williams and Wilkins, PO Box 23291, Baltimore, MD 21203-9990

Irvine Perry, Sherry
1992 AIDS, Blindness, and Rehabilitation: From Home Experience to the Workplace RE:view
    XXIII(Winter)4:186-189

Kiester, Edwin Jr.
1990 AIDS & Vision Loss New York, NY: American Foundation for the Blind

Vocational Rehabilitation Services to Persons with H.I.V. (AIDS), Research and Training Center, Publications, Department AB, University of Wisconsin-Stout, Menomonie, WI 54751

REFERRAL RESOURCES

Organizations

CDC National AIDS Hotline
(800) 342-AIDS   (800) 344-7432 (Spanish)   (800) 243-7889 (TT)

A 24 hour hot-line that provides information about HIV transmission and prevention, HIV testing and treatment, referrals, and educational materials. Special resources are available for minorities and women. Spanish information specialists are available 8:00 a.m. to 2:00 a.m. Eastern Time and a Spanish recording is available from 2:00 a.m. to 8:00 a.m.

AIDS, Blindness and Low Vision: A Guide for Service Providers
by Mary Ann Lang, Carol Sussman-Skalka, and Margaret Galligan
Lighthouse Low Vision Products
36-02 Northern Boulevard
Long Island City, NY 11101
(800) 453-4925   (718) 937-6959   FAX (718) 786-0437

Based on the experiences Lighthouse staff have had in working with patients with AIDS, this booklet provides information on rehabilitation for patients with AIDS and guidelines for establishing an AIDS program. Single copy, FREE; multiple copies, $1.00 each

ALBINISM

Albinism is a hereditary condition in which the normal amount of pigment is lacking in the eyes, hair, and/or skin. When it is caused by a deficiency of the enzyme tyrosinase, it is called tyrosinase-negative or complete albinism. Light sensitivity varies from mild difficulty to photophobia. Other visual characteristics include decreased acuity, strabismus, and nystagmus (involuntary, rapid eye movements). Hats, sunglasses, and visors help to minimize glare.

Tyrosinase-positive albinism, or incomplete albinism, does not cause the dramatic lack of pigment in skin, eyes, and hair. It is more difficult to diagnose because the symptoms are less evident and most individuals with this type of albinism function as normally sighted (Faye: 1984).

It is important that families receive genetic counseling to understand the hereditary patterns of their particular condition. Organizations of people with albinism provide emotional support and education and deal with issues of appearance. Individuals with reduced acuity will benefit from rehabilitation and low vision aids. Children with albinism may need special accommodations in the classroom, such as LARGE PRINT books, seating in the front of the room, and the services of a vision teacher (See Chapter 5, "Special Population Groups," Children and Adolescents).

References

Faye, Eleanor
1984 Clinical Low Vision Boston, MA: Little, Brown and Company

Facts About Albinism
by James Haefemeyer, Richard King, and Bonnie Leroy
International Albinism Center
Box 485 UMIC, University of Minnesota
420 Delaware Street SE
Minneapolis, MN 55455
(612) 624-0144

Answers most commonly asked questions about albinism, $3.00.

National Organization for Albinism and Hypopigmentation (NOAH)
1500 Locust Street, Suite 1816
Philadelphia, PA 19102
(800) 473-2310   (215) 545-2322

Support organization with chapters across U.S. Newsletter,"NOAH News," is published in LARGE PRINT in English and Spanish, twice a year. Membership, $10.00. Publishes "The Student with Albinism in the Regular Classroom," a book that describes the special needs of children with albinism and suggests adaptations for classroom and nonclassroom activities. LARGE PRINT. $3.50

CORNEAL DISORDERS

Although corneal diseases and injuries are responsible for only about six percent of the cases of legal blindness in the U.S., they are the primary cause of blindness worldwide (National Eye Institute: 1987). Major corneal diseases and conditions seen in the U.S. include infectious forms such as herpes simplex; ocular surface problems such as keratoconjunctivitis sicca, often associated with Sjogren's syndrome (see "Sjogren's Syndrome" below); corneal dystrophies; and trauma. The use of extended wear contact lenses has been implicated as a cause of corneal infections; extensive public education campaigns have stressed the importance of proper care and cleaning of contact lenses.

Corneal transplants, while successful in many cases, still pose problems of immunologic rejection. Clinical studies are evaluating graft reactions and suggest that tissue typing for better matches, control of vascularization through laser therapy or medication, and controlling the immune system, may achieve higher rates of success (National Eye Institute: 1987).

Individuals who have had unsuccessful corneal transplants should be referred for rehabilitation services. Support groups may provide important emotional support for individuals dealing with transplant rejection.

References

National Eye Institute
1987 Annual Report

REFERRAL RESOURCES

Eye Bank Association of America
1001 Connecticut Avenue, NW, Suite 601
Washington, DC 20036-5504
(202) 775-4999

An organization of eye banks in the United States, Canada, and Mexico which provide tissue for corneal transplants. Funds research projects and promotes eye and tissue donation through posters, brochures, and videotapes.

National Ambassadors for Corneal Transplant
PO Box 342
Painted Post, NY 14870-0342
(800) 462-1011

Provides support to individuals considering a corneal transplant through a peer counseling program and a LARGE PRINT booklet, A New Outlook: Your Corneal Transplant, $5.00.

Tissue Banks International (TBI)
815 Park Avenue
Baltimore, MD 21201
(410) 752-3800   FAX (410) 727-3843   Tissue request (800) 858-2020

A network of eye banks throughout the U.S., TBI coordinates the donation of tissue. Provides public information. Surgeons may contact the tissue request number seven days a week.

Monocular vision is most frequently caused by trauma or diseases that require removal of an eye. Ocular trauma may be caused by sports injuries; use of fireworks, motorized gardening equipment such as lawnmowers, trimmers and edgers; and automobile accidents. Retinoblastoma, a cancer that requires removal of the eye, is the most common primary tumor of the eye in children (American Cancer Society: 1992). In adults, ocular melanoma is the most common primary eye cancer (National Cancer Institute: 1992).

When an individual's eye is surgically enucleated, it is usually replaced by a prosthesis. An ocularist works with the ophthalmologist and the patient in prescribing, selecting, and fitting a prosthesis. Plastic surgery may be required to repair the eye socket and surrounding tissue. A properly fitted prosthesis will allow satisfactory eye movement and appear as similar to the remaining eye as possible.

A major functional limitation of monocular vision is the loss of depth perception. The visual field is reduced and visual processing becomes disorganized. Individuals must learn to move more slowly, to move their heads to compensate for visual field loss, and to develop techniques for judging distance. Optical aids such as magnifiers and monocular telescopes, LARGE PRINT, and good lighting are all useful in adapting to monocular vision. Individuals with monocular vision should wear safety glasses to protect their remaining vision.

Many individuals find it useful to speak to others who have experienced enucleation; therefore, referral to a self-help group may be beneficial.

References

American Cancer Society
1992 "Retinoblastoma" Cancer Response System (800) ACS-2345

Brady, Frank B.
1988 <u>A Singular View: The Art of Seeing with One Eye</u> Frank B. Brady Author/Publisher PO Box 4653, Annapolis, MD

National Cancer Institute
1992 <u>Melanoma Research Report</u> National Cancer Institute, Office of Cancer Communications, Bethesda, MD 20892

Singular Vision Outreach
1992 "An Eye on the Future" Singular Vision Outreach, PO Box 1451, Maryland Heights, MO 63043

PROFESSIONAL ORGANIZATIONS

American Society of Ocularists
244 East Park Avenue, #103
Lake Wales, FL 33853
(813) 676-2737

Professional organization for ocularists. Publishes "You and Your Ocularist," a guide for choosing a prosthetic eye. FREE

REFERRAL RESOURCES

Singular Vision Outreach (SVOR)
PO Box 1451
Maryland Heights, MO 63040
(314) 453-9905

Assists individuals adjusting to monocular vision and their families through information and referral, support, and consultation. Educates the general public about eye safety and works with health professionals. Publishes newsletter, "An Eye on the Future," and "Driving Tips for Monocular Individuals," FREE. Membership, individual $15.00; family, $25.00.

MULTIPLE SCLEROSIS

Multiple sclerosis (MS) is a chronic disease which affects the central nervous system. Individuals with multiple sclerosis generally experience attacks and remissions of symptoms. The visual symptoms may include blurred vision in one eye, double vision, or nystagmus (involuntary, rapid eye movements). Visual symptoms are often transitory and improve or clear within a few months. Color vision is also affected by multiple sclerosis, because the nerve fibers responsible for determining color are disrupted.

Optic neuritis, which recurs with the attacks and remissions of the disease itself, may produce a large blind spot, or central scotoma, interfering with central vision. Lechtenberg (1988) reports that up to 90% of young people who develop optic neuritis are diagnosed as having multiple sclerosis at a later date.

The functional implications of central vision loss include restriction in activities such as driving and reading. Double vision affects reading, walking, and other movement; patching one eye may make the individual more comfortable.

Although individuals with transitory vision problems may not be eligible for services from public agencies, referrals to private agencies may enable these individuals to remain independent and retain their employment. Special transportation services and computer equipment with LARGE PRINT or speech output may prove useful.

References

Lechtenberg, Richard
1988 Multiple Sclerosis Fact Book Philadelphia, PA: F.A. Davis Company

REFERRAL RESOURCES

National Multiple Sclerosis Society
733 Third Avenue
New York, NY 10017-3288
(800) 624-8236   (212) 986-3240   FAX (212) 986-7981

Provides information, emotional support, and practical assistance through more than 150 local chapters and branches. Publishes a series of "Fact & Issues" articles, including "Insight into Eyesight," LARGE PRINT. Quarterly magazine, "Inside MS," (also available on audio-cassette). Membership, $20.00

Talking Books and Multiple Sclerosis
National Library Service for the Blind and Physically Handicapped (NLS)
1291 Taylor Street, NW
Washington, DC 20542
(800) 424-8567 or 8572 (Reference Section)
(800) 424-9100 (to receive application)
(202) 707-5100   FAX (202) 707-0712

Describes the eligibility requirements for individuals with multiple sclerosis. FREE

Understanding Multiple Sclerosis: A New Handbook for Families
by Robert Shuman and Janice Schwartz
Macmillan Publishing Company, Riverside, NJ

Discusses the role of the family, adolescents with multiple sclerosis, and lists resources. $19.95, plus $1.50 shipping and handling.

Retinopathy of prematurity (ROP) involves the growth of abnormal blood vessels and scar tissue in the vitreous and retinal detachments in low birth weight premature infants. First observed in the 1940's, this condition was originally called retrolental fibroplasia (RLF) and attributed to the use of excessive oxygen in the incubators. This single cause is no longer supported (Zierler: 1988); other factors which have been implicated are deficiency in vitamin A and E, low oxygen and high carbon dioxide blood levels, and other metabolic factors (Repka: 1989). Most researchers agree that prematurity itself and low birth weight are primary contributors to retinopathy of prematurity.

Retinopathy of prematurity should be detected in the neonatal unit through ophthalmoscopic examination of the infant's dilated eyes. Although in some infants, the abnormal blood vessels shrink and do not affect vision, in others the retina may become distorted or detached, resulting in varying degrees of vision loss. Researchers caution that children whose retinopathy of prematurity has regressed may be at risk for other eye conditions such as amblyopia, strabismus, and refractive disorders (Kalina: 1988). Long term complications observed in older children and young adults include retinal detachment and narrow-angle glaucoma (Repka: 1989). Both health care and rehabilitation professionals should suggest regular ophthalmological examinations for individuals with retinopathy of prematurity.

Clinical trials to evaluate the effects of cryotherapy, in which peripheral areas of the retina are frozen in order to slow or reverse development of abnormal blood vessels and scar tissue, have concluded that this treatment is effective in a large number of cases that have reached a threshold level of the disease (Cryotherapy for Retinopathy of Prematurity Cooperative Group: 1990). This controlled study found that just over half of eyes that had not received cryotherapy had unfavorable outcomes compared to 31.1% of the treated eyes. In order to compare the long term results in treated and untreated eyes, the study is continuing to follow the subjects until they are six years old (Palmer: 1990).

Vitrectomy, a surgical means of clearing the vitreous of scar tissue and treating retinal detachment, has not proven to be as successful (Quinn et al.: 1991). Some investigators have found that Vitamin E is an effective treatment for preventing retinopathy of prematurity (Quinn et al.: 1990). A pilot study of laser photocoagulation to treat retinopathy of prematurity suggests that this treatment mode results in a favorable outcome when compared to untreated eyes, although more research on this method is needed (Landers et al.: 1992).

Health professionals such as the neonatologist, ophthalmologist, and pediatrician must provide coordinated medical care to the infant with retinopathy of prematurity; they must also care for the child's parents. Because low birth weight babies often have multiple disabilities, a number of health care and rehabilitation professionals are likely to provide care for the baby. All service providers involved in the care and discharge of infants with retinopathy of prematurity should be aware of the risks of this condition and should make appropriate referrals for ophthalmic care. Teplin (1988) recommends that professionals discuss the parents' questions and concerns; recognize that early intervention and parent education are important for normal development; and recognize that the physician must take the initiative in making referrals to supportive agencies and resources. Teplin's list of ten roles for physicians to promote optimal development of blind children and infants may be used as guidelines by any health care or rehabilitation professional. Failure to make referrals causes the family to "flounder needlessly, while the infant misses valuable opportunities for cognitive, motor, and emotional development" (Teplin: 1988:302).   Once children with retinopathy of prematurity enter school, teachers and other school staff should be informed about the condition and the risk of developing other eye disorders, so that they may report any unusual visual behavior to the parents.

Chapter 5,   "Special Population Groups," Children and Adolescents,   discusses educational needs, benefits, resources, and literature available for health and rehabilitation professionals who work with children who are visually impaired or blind.

References

Cryotherapy for Retinopathy of Prematurity Cooperative Group
1990 "Multicenter Trial of Cryotherapy for Retinopathy of Prematurity" Archives of Ophthalmology 108(February):195-204

Kalina, Robert E.
1988 "Diagnosis and Early Follow-Up of Retinopathy of Prematurity" pp. 185-191 in John T. Flynn and Dale L. Phelps (eds.) Retinopathy of Prematurity: Problem and Challenge New York, NY: Alan R. Liss, Inc.

Landers, Maurice, B., Cynthia A. Toth, Christopher Semple, and Lawrence S. Morse
1992 "Treatment of Retinopathy of Prematurity with Argon Laser Photocoagulation" Archives of Ophthalmology 110(January):44-47

Palmer, Earl A.
1990 "Results of U.S. Randomized Clinical Trial of Cryotherapy for ROP Documenta Ophthalmologica 74:245-51

Quinn, Graham E., Velma Dobson, Charles C. Barr, Barry R. Davis, John T. Flynn, Earl A. Palmer, Joseph Robertson, and Michael T. Trese
1991 "Visual Acuity in Infants after Vitrectomy for Severe Retinopathy of Prematurity" Ophthalmology 98(January):5-13

Quinn, Graham E., Lois Johnson, Chari Otis, David B. Schaffer, and Frank W. Bowen
1990 "Incidence, Severity and Time Course of ROP in a Randomized Clinical Trial of Vitamin E Prophylaxis" Documenta Ophthalmologica 74:223-28

Repka, Michael X.
1989 "Update on Retinopathy of Prematurity" Future Reflections 8:3:29-31

Teplin, Stuart W.
1988 "Development of the Blind Infant and Child with Retinopathy of Prematurity: The Physician's Role in Intervention," pp. 301-323 in John T. Flynn and Dale L. Phelps (eds.) Retinopathy of Prematurity: Problem and Challenge New York, NY: Alan R. Liss, Inc.

Zierler, Sally
1988 "Causes of Retinopathy of Prematurity: An Epidemiologic Perspective" pp. 23-33 in John T. Flynn and Dale L. Phelps (eds.) Retinopathy of Prematurity: Problem and Challenge New York, NY: Alan R. Liss, Inc.

SJOGREN'S SYNDROME

Sjogren's syndrome is a chronic autoimmune condition characterized by dryness of the eyes, mouth, and skin caused by the destruction of the lymph glands (National Institute of Arthritis and Musculoskeletal and Skin Diseases: 1988). If the cornea is disturbed, vision problems may result. Sjogren's syndrome may be a primary disease or it may accompany rheumatic disease, often rheumatoid arthritis. According to the National Institute of Arthritis and Musculoskeletal and Skin Diseases, individuals with Sjogren's syndrome may have an increased risk for developing lymphomas, inflammatory blood vessel disease, and nervous system dysfunction.

Artificial tears and eye drops, mouth rinses and fluids, and moisturizing lotions are used to treat this syndrome. Medications which may be prescribed to relieve symptoms include aspirin, nonsteroidal anti-inflammatory drugs, and corticosteroids (NIAMS: 1986).

References

National Arthritis and Musculoskeletal and Skin Diseases Information Clearinghouse (NIAMS)
1986 Patient Education Resources Bethesda, MD

National Institute of Arthritis and Musculoskeletal and Skin Diseases
1988 Arthritis, Rheumatic Diseases, and Related Disorders Bethesda, MD: National Institutes of Health

Harris, Elaine K.
1992 "The Self-Help Approach to Sjogren's Syndrome" pp. 205-13 in Alfred H. Katz et al. (eds.) Self-Help: Concepts and Applications Philadelphia, PA: The Charles Press

National Arthritis and Musculoskeletal and Skin Diseases Information Clearinghouse
1987 Sjogren's Syndrome: Professional Education Materials Bethesda, MD

REFERRAL RESOURCES

Arthritis Foundation
1314 Spring Street, NW
Atlanta, GA 30309
(800) 283-7800   (404) 872-7100

Publishes "Sjogren's Syndrome," a brochure which explains causes, symptoms, diagnosis, and treatment for this related condition.   Membership fee of $15.00, includes chapter newsletter and magazine, "Arthritis Today."

National Arthritis and Musculoskeletal and Skin Diseases Information Clearinghouse
Box AMS
Bethesda, MD 20892
(301) 468-3235

Publishes annotated bibliography, "Sjogren's Syndrome: Patient Education Materials." $2.00.

National Sjogren's Syndrome Association
3201 West Evans Drive
Phoenix, AZ 85023
(800) 395-6772   (602) 993-7227

Provides information to patients and professionals through support groups and conferences throughout the U.S. Membership, $20.00, includes quarterly Patient Education Series and newsletter, "Sjogren's Digest." Publishes "Sjogren's Syndrome: The Sneaky Arthritis." U.S., $12.50; foreign, $14.00.

Sjogren's Syndrome Foundation
382 Main Street
Port Washington, NY 11050
(516) 767-2866

Contact persons in many U.S. cities, Canada, and abroad. Publishes newsletter, "The Moisture Seekers," and "The Sjogren's Syndrome Handbook," a guide for living more comfortably with this chronic illness. $19.95, plus $2.50 shipping and handling; shipping to Canada, $7.00. Membership, U.S., $25.00; Canada, $35.00.

STROKE-RELATED VISION LOSS

Individuals who have had a stroke may lose some of their visual field; a loss of right field vision in both eyes is called "right hemiplegia;" loss of left visual field in both eyes is called "left hemiplegia." Individuals with hemiplegia must learn to turn their heads to compensate for the field loss. Some individuals find that using a patch over one eye helps to reduce spatial problems due to hemiplegia.

Because strokes may cause a multiplicity of impairments, a number of professional service providers are involved in the rehabilitation process. These include ophthalmologists, neurologists, occupational and physical therapists, audiologists and speech pathologists, and rehabilitation counselors and teachers. It is useful to have one professional take the role of case manager or coordinator to ensure that the treatments and therapies recommended by the various professionals are coordinated and do not overburden the patient or client.

REFERRAL RESOURCES

Organizations

American Heart Association (AHA)
7320 Greenville Avenue
Dallas, TX 75231
(214) 750-3500

Promotes research and education, sponsors stroke clubs, and publishes public education brochures. Local affiliates. Publications that discuss stroke-related vision loss include "Stroke: Why Do They Behave That Way?" "Recovering from a Stroke," and "Do It Yourself Again." Single copies FREE. Also available from affiliates.

Courage Stroke Network
3915 Golden Valley Road
Golden Valley, MN 55422
(800) 553-6321   (612) 588-0811

Offers information and referral, peer counseling, and education through 700 independent stroke groups in the U.S. Newsletter, "Stroke Connection." Membership, $7.00 FREE catalogue.

Heart and Stroke Foundation of Canada
160 George Street, Suite 200
Ottawa, Ontario K1N 9M2 Canada
(613) 237-4361

Conducts research; provides professional and public education through provincial divisions and chapters. FREE publications list.

National Stroke Association
300 East Hampden Avenue, Suite 240
Englewood, CO 80110-2622
(303) 762-9922   FAX (303) 762-1190

Assists individuals with stroke and educates their families, physicians, and the general public about stroke. Membership, $10.00, includes quarterly newsletter, "Be Stroke Smart." Also available "The Road Ahead: A Stroke Recovery Guide." $14.50

Stroke Recovery Association
585 Trethewey Drive
Toronto, Ontario M6M 4B8 Canada
(416) 614-3271

Provides information and emotional support to people who have had strokes and their families. Monthly magazine, "Phoenix." Membership, $15.00 per family, Canadian funds

Publications and Tapes

After a Stroke
Resources for Rehabilitation
33 Bedford Street, Suite 19A
Lexington, MA 02173
(617) 862-6455   FAX (617) 861-7517

Designed for distribution by professionals, this LARGE PRINT (18 point bold type) publication includes information on how to obtain services; organizations; publications; and assistive devices. Minimum purchase, 25 copies. $2.00 per copy. Discounts available for purchases of 100 or more copies. See order form on last page of book.

Resources for Elders with Disabilities
Resources for Rehabilitation
33 Bedford Street, Suite 19A
Lexington, MA 02173
(617) 862-6455   FAX (617) 861-7517

A LARGE PRINT resource directory that describes services and products that help elders with disabilities to function independently. Includes chapters on stroke, vision loss, hearing loss, arthritis, diabetes, Parkinson's disease, falls, and osteoporosis. Updated biennially. $39.95 plus $5.00 shipping and handling

SPECIAL POPULATION GROUPS

CHILDREN AND ADOLESCENTS

When parents learn that their child is visually impaired or blind, they are often overwhelmed by their own emotional responses as well as the pressures of providing the child with the best possible medical and rehabilitation services. At a time when they often feel guilty, frightened about their child's future, and depressed, they must learn about a new system of services and how to integrate these services into their family life.

Parents are rarely prepared for this situation, unless by chance they have friends or family members who have dealt with a similar condition in their own family. A variety of factors influence families' coping mechanisms, including educational level of parents, financial status, personality characteristics of family members, and the availability of services to help the child. Although some families may break up as a result of the stress caused by having a child with a disability or chronic condition, others become closer (Shapiro: 1983).

Because parents experience such intense emotional reactions to a child's visual impairment or blindness, counseling to help them cope with their own emotions will contribute to their ability to help the child. Such counseling may be available from medical professionals, social workers or psychologists, rehabilitation counselors, and other parents in similar situations. Talking with other parents either in private or at a parent support group helps parents learn that their emotional responses are normal.

Stress factors which affect the families of children who are visually impaired or blind include financial problems, often caused by limitations of health insurance coverage; lack of information about medical and community services available; and the need to restructure the family itself. It is wise to schedule visits to physicians and other service providers' offices so that parents can share the responsibility for the child's care.

When other children are in the family, the situation is compounded by the need to preserve a sense of normalcy and at the same time help the child who has a disability. Siblings may be jealous of the attention paid to the child who is visually impaired or blind. Local agencies that serve children who are visually impaired or blind provide help and support for parents and other family members. Some offer parent support groups, where members learn from each others' experiences about how to cope emotionally as well as how to find the resources to help their children develop.

As the child develops and enters new environments, it is important for his or her peers to be educated about visual impairment or blindness. Children must learn that individuals who

Rehabilitation Resource Manual: VISION Lexington, MA: Resources for Rehabilitation copyright 1993

are different should not be viewed negatively. Children who do not have disabilities should be encouraged to ask adults questions about disabilities. They should be told that teasing will hurt the other child's feelings. Disability awareness programs in schools, religious organizations, and youth groups offer an opportunity to educate children about a specific disability. The "Kids on the Block" programs (see "ORGANIZATIONS" section below) enable children to simulate an experience with blindness and related conditions such as diabetes, thereby encouraging understanding and acceptance.

Visual impairment and blindness in children, whether it is congenital or it occurs later in childhood, affects neurological development; reflexes; emotional development; and the development of language (Jan and Robinson: 1989). A recent study found that the majority of infants who were visually impaired (birth to three years) in one county had multiple handicaps (Williamson et al.: 1987). In order to ensure that infants and children receive the services that they need from a variety of health care and rehabilitation professionals, ophthalmologists should be in contact with pediatricians as well as the local school system or the state department of special education to obtain information about services available from governmental agencies. Ophthalmology departments in children's hospitals may have special resources and programs for children with visual impairments.

Children from birth through two years of age who have developmental delays due to visual impairments are eligible for special instruction through early intervention programs. State departments of education may apply for federal funding for special services for infants and toddlers with disabilities. One of the requirements for receiving these funds is that a central directory of intervention services and resources be produced (U.S. Department of Education: 1988).

Children may receive instruction in subjects such as typing or braille in a specially equipped resource room or on an as-needed basis through consultation with the regular classroom teacher. Schools which serve large numbers of children who are visually impaired or blind employ full-time teachers to provide these services. Schools with few students who are visually impaired or blind employ itinerant vision teachers, who often work for a collaborative of area schools.

Many children with multiple disabilities including visual impairment or blindness are served by public school programs. However, some of these students may require a concentrated program that results in placement in a residential facility. Residential facilities may also offer a combination of educational resources needed by the gifted youngster who is visually impaired or blind, or these services may be available in gifted-student programs in public schools.

State agencies serving individuals who are visually impaired or blind often offer special services such as home visits, infant-toddler programs, counseling for parents, information and referral, summer camp funding, after-school programs, and other supplementary services (See "Appendix A: State Agencies for Individuals Who Are Visually Impaired or Blind"). In addition, some private agencies have been established for the specific purpose of providing services to children who are visually impaired or blind and to their families.

Although numerous professionals may be involved in helping children who are visually impaired or blind, ultimately it is the parents' responsibility to ensure that their child receives optimal medical care, rehabilitation, and education. Gliedman and Roth make several suggestions to help parents achieve this goal, including monitoring the child's progress closely; keeping copies of the child's records; keeping records of visits with professionals, including dates, who was present, and what was said; learning as much as possible about the child's condition; listening to the child when he or she expresses individual needs; and staying in touch with the child's teacher (1980: pp. 184-185)

LAWS AND EDUCATION

The enactment of the *Education of the Handicapped Act* (P.L. 94-142) in 1975 broke ground for the expansion of educational services for children with disabilities and established legal rights for these children to obtain an appropriate education from the public school system. In 1990, the name of the Education of the Handicapped Act was changed to the *Individuals with Disabilities Education Act*, referred to as IDEA (P.L. 101-476). The law requires that states provide all children with disabilities an appropriate public education in the least restrictive setting. Special education services provided in public school classrooms, at home, and in hospitals and institutions are included. Related services that states must provide include transportation; physical and occupational therapy; and psychological services (U.S. Department of Education: 1988).

In order for states to receive federal funding for programs for children with disabilities, the state department of education must establish a plan and procedures for providing these services and require that local educational agencies maintain individualized education plans (IEP's) for each child served. Federal funds are allocated to states based on the number of children served. In the 1986-87 school year, 4.4 million children and youths (ages 3 to 21) received services mandated by this law and by the Education Consolidation and Improvement Act - State Operated Programs. Of the students served, 27,049 were visually impaired (0.7% of those receiving services) and another 1,766 were deaf-blind (0.1%) (Kraus and Stoddard: 1989).

In addition, the federal law has mandated that regional resource centers be established to provide technical assistance to professional educators who provide services for children and youth with disabilities. These centers may be operated by a college or university, state or local education agency, or private nonprofit organization that has received a federal grant for this purpose. The state educational agency is required to publish a listing of the resource centers in the state. Training centers to help parents of children with disabilities interact more effectively with professionals were mandated by the 1990 and 1991 amendments to IDEA.

The *Education of the Handicapped Act Amendments of 1983* (P.L. 98-199) expanded the incentives to local and state governments to provide equal educational opportunities in preschool, early intervention, and transition programs. The *Education of the Handicapped Act Amendments of 1986* (P.L. 99-457) lowered the eligibility for special education services to age three and established the Handicapped Infant and Toddler Programs (birth to age three). These programs provide early intervention services to infants and toddlers who have been diagnosed with physical or mental conditions for which there is a high probability of developmental delay (Center for Special Education Technology: 1991). States are required to develop a comprehensive, statewide, interagency service delivery system by their fifth year of participation in the program (National Information Center for Children and Youth with Disabilities: 1991).

Under the provisions of the various Acts cited above, the special education teacher, health care providers, and the parents work together to develop an Individualized Education Plan (IEP), which specifies educational goals, courses of instruction, special equipment, and other services to be provided. The vision teacher serves as the "case manager" and recommends the services of other team members such as orientation and mobility instructors, counselors, and speech and language therapists. The IEP is based on the results of an individualized evaluation and assessment of the child. Schools are required to notify parents in writing any time a decision is made related to the identification of the child's disability, educational needs, development of the IEP, or placement in a special or regular program. Parents have the right to appeal if they disagree with the school's decision and may arrange for an independent evaluation of their child.

Adolescents who are visually impaired or blind have special needs as they consider career goals and higher education. Vocational education offers students a combination of classroom instruction and practical job experience to develop the occupational skills needed in the labor market. Vocational education is available in high schools, community colleges, and technical institutes. The *Carl D. Perkins Vocational and Applied Technology Education Act* (P.L. 101-392) provides increased resources to achieve the academic and occupational skills necessary for employment in high technology. Individuals with disabilities are included in this mandate.

Section 504 of the Rehabilitation Act of 1973 prohibits any institution that receives federal funds from discriminating against people with disabilities. Since virtually all postsecondary institutions receive federal funds, they are required to comply with the regulations developed for the enforcement of Section 504. Students who qualify for admission into postsecondary education programs must be provided with the services that they need to complete their education (Bowe: 1987). Most universities, colleges, and community colleges have established special offices to serve students with disabilities. For students who are visually impaired or blind, these services may include volunteer readers, special equipment to enlarge the print size of reading materials, or specially adapted computer equipment. Most universities, colleges, and community colleges have established special offices to serve students with disabilities. Sources of financial assistance for postsecondary students with disabilities are listed below under "Financial Aid for Postsecondary Education."

Children with disabilities may be eligible for *Social Security* benefits. The Social Security Administration can advise parents whether their child is eligible for medical or cash benefits. Eligibility criteria have recently been changed as a result of a court decision (Parker: 1991). Children must be disabled and their families must meet a financial means test. Many children who were denied benefits during the period 1980 to 1990 may now be eligible and may also receive retroactive payment for benefits that were previously denied.

References

Bowe, Frank G.
1987 "Section 504: 10 Years Later" American Rehabilitation (April/May/June):2-3;23-24

Center for Special Education Technology
1991 "Update: 1990 Demographic Data" The Marketplace: Report on Technology in Special Education 4:1

Gliedman, John and William Roth
1980 The Unexpected Minority: Handicapped Children in America New York, NY: Harcourt Brace Jovanovich

Jan, James E. and Geoffrey C. Robinson
1989 "A Multidisciplinary Program for Visually Impaired Children and Youth" International Ophthalmology Clinics 29(Spring):32-36

Kraus, Lewis E. and Susan Stoddard
1989 Chartbook on Disability in the United States An InfoUse Report Washington, DC: National Institute on Disability and Rehabilitation Research

National Information Center for Children and Youth with Disabilities
1991 "The Education of Children and Youth with Special Needs: What Do the Laws Say?" NICHCY News Digest I:1

Parker, Susan
1991 "Changes in the Way Social Security Evaluates Claims for Childhood Disability Benefits" Journal of Disability Policy Studies 2(2):77-86

Shapiro, Johanna
1983 "Family Reactions and Coping Strategies in Response to the Physically Ill or Handicapped Child: A Review" Social Science and Medicine 17:14:913-931

U.S. Department of Education
1988 <u>Summary of Existing Legislation Affection Persons with Disabilities</u> Washington, DC: Office of Special Education and Rehabilitative Services, Clearinghouse on the Handicapped, Publication No. E-88-22014

Williamson, W. Daniel, Murdina M. Desmond, Leora P. Andrew, and Rose Hicks
1987 "Visually Impaired Infants in the 1980's" <u>Clinical Pediatrics</u> 26(May): 241-244

Jean Raleigh: A Student with Low Vision

Jean Raleigh is a nine year old who is visually impaired due to albinism. Her acuity is 20/80, which has enabled her to read the large print found in textbooks used in the early grades. She is entering the fourth grade in a new school following her family's move during the summer. Since textbooks in upper grades are generally printed in smaller type, this is the first year that Jean may need special reading materials.

Jean's classroom teacher, Mr. Richard Taggart, has been advised of her visual status and is concerned about meeting her special needs. Jean's parents and school officials, including the principal, Mr. Taggart, the gym teacher, and a special vision teacher, Ms Roundtree, are meeting to develop her Individualized Education Plan (IEP). Jean's parents are concerned that the IEP may not be approved and signed in time for the opening of school. Therefore, Ms Roundtree has advised Mr. Taggart to call the state department of special education vision resources library to request a set of textbooks in large print.

Ms Roundtree has also suggested that Jean sit near the front of the class in order to see the blackboard and that Mr. Taggart repeat verbally whatever he writes on the board. Since worksheets are duplicated by purple spirit masters, Ms Roundtree has recommended that Jean use a yellow acetate theme cover to slip over the sheets. The purple print appears black under the yellow acetate, providing much better contrast for easier reading.

At the meeting, the gym teacher expresses doubts about Jean's participation in physical education activities. She feels that Jean may have problems with a sport such as baseball, but that she should be encouraged to participate in swimming and dancing. Jean's parents want their daughter to participate in as many activities as possible. To resolve this conflict, Ms Roundtree suggests that Jean's ophthalmologist submit a report to the school indicating what activities are permissible and that this information be shared with the gym teacher. Ms Roundtree also suggests that Jean have a low vision evaluation in order to determine her current acuity. Jean's parents concur with these suggestions.

Continued on next page

In a letter to Dr. Frances Allbright, Ms Roundtree requests the ophthalmologist's advice and suggests a referral for a low vision evaluation. Dr. Allbright works with an optometrist, Dr. Dean Whalom, who is able to schedule an appointment prior to the start of school. After the low vision evaluation, Dr. Whalom prescribes a monocular for distance viewing, large print software for computer work, and a magnifier with a light for reading texts. At her age, Jean is having fun showing these aids to her new friends, who think that these devices are "pretty neat."

Following their respective examinations, Dr. Allbright and Dr. Whalom send a joint report to the school and to Jean's parents, indicating that Jean's acuity has remained stable at 20/80 and describing the aids that have been prescribed for specific activities. Although Jean need not be restricted in her physical education activities, they recommend that she wear safety glasses during gym class.

(In the listings below, telephone numbers have symbols V for voice and TT for text telephone where organizations have published this information.)

American Council on Rural Special Education (ACRES)
Miller Hall 359
Western Washington University
Bellingham, WA 98225
(206) 676-3576

National membership organization for educators who serve individuals with disabilities in rural areas. Membership, $45.00. Publishes "Rural Special Education Quarterly," "RuraLink," and the "Journal of Rural and Small Schools." Provides scholarships for practicing rural teachers who work with students with disabilities.

American Printing House for the Blind (APH)
1839 Frankfort Avenue
PO Box 6085
Louisville, KY 40206-0095
(800) 223-1839   (502) 895-2405   FAX (502) 895-1509

Publishes elementary and secondary school textbooks in LARGE PRINT, recorded format, or braille. Sells special aids and tools for students and adults with vision loss through the "Instructional Aids, Tools, and Supplies" catalog, FREE.

Association on Higher Education and Disability (AHEAD)
PO Box 21192
Columbus, OH 43221-0192
(614) 488-4972 (V/TT)   FAX (614) 488-1174

Promotes the full participation of individuals with disabilities in postsecondary education. Provides ADA compliance assistance to universities through publications and ADA Hot Line (800) 247-7752. Members receive the "Journal of Postsecondary Education and Disability" and "ALERT" Newsletter. Special interest groups focus on specific disabilities such as visual impairment and blindness, technology, and other topics.

Children's SSI Campaign
Mental Health Law Project
1101 15th Street, NW, Suite 1212
Washington, DC 20005
(202) 467-5730   (202) 467-4232 (TT)   FAX (202) 223-0409

Provides an "Action Kit" for professionals to use in community outreach for children with disabilities who may be eligible for Social Security Benefits, FREE. Will answer questions about eligibility. Publishes "The Advocate's Guide to SSI for Children,"a manual that helps service providers understand the application and appeals procedures for financial and disability based eligibility. $75.00 (10% discount for prepaid orders)

Council for Exceptional Children (CEC)
1920 Association Drive
Reston, VA 22091-1589
(703) 620-3660 (V/TT)   FAX (703) 264-9494

A professional membership organization that works toward improving the quality of education for children who have disabilities or are gifted. CEC's Division for the Visually Handicapped publishes its own newsletter four times per year. Publishes two journals that are included with membership: "Teaching Exceptional Children," (subscription for nonmembers, U.S., $30.00; foreign, $35.00) and "Exceptional Children" (subscription for nonmembers, U.S., $45.00; foreign, $51.00). Holds annual conference. Manages ERIC Clearinghouse on Handicapped and Gifted, which contains abstracts of published literature. CEC will perform custom computer searches of its databases; phone (703) 264-9474.

Lighthouse National Center for Vision and Child Development
800 Second Avenue
New York, NY 10017
(800) 334-5497 (V/TT)   (212) 808-0077   FAX (212) 808-0110

Provides training for service providers who work with children and their families and technical assistance for schools, day care centers, health facilities, and other organizations. Conducts research related to child development and vision loss.

National Association of State Directors of Special Education (NASDSE)
2021 K Street, NW, Suite 315
Washington, DC 20036-1003
(202) 296-1800

A coalition of state directors of special education. Published the entire text of the Individuals with Disabilities Education Act, including the 1990 amendments. $15.00

National Center for Youth with Disabilities (NCYD)
Box 721 UMHC
Harvard Street at East River Road
Minneapolis, MN 55455
(800) 333-6293   (612) 626-2825   (612) 624-3939 (TT)
FAX (612) 626-2134

Provides information and technical assistance on the needs of adolescents and young adults with chronic illnesses and disabilities. National resource library available through computer database. "CYDLINE Reviews" are a series of annotated bibliographies on topics related to youth with disabilities; prices vary with content. Quarterly newsletter, "Connections," FREE.

Rehabilitation Engineering Center of the Smith Kettlewell Eye Research Institute
2232 Webster Street
San Francisco, CA 94115
(415) 561-1619   FAX (415) 561-1610

A federally funded center that develops and tests new technology for individuals who are visually impaired, blind, or deaf-blind, with special projects related to children and educational aids.

Sibling Information Network
University Affiliated Program
University of Connecticut
991 Main Street, Suite 3A
East Hartford, CT 06108
(203) 282-7050

Clearinghouse for information, literature, and research about siblings and other issues of families of individuals with disabilities. Quarterly "Sibling Information Network Newsletter," includes SIBPAGE, an insert written by and for siblings, ages 5 to 15, FREE.

TASH: The Association for Persons with Severe Handicaps
11201 Greenwood Avenue North
Seattle, WA 98133
(206) 361-8870   (206) 361-0133 (TT)   FAX (206) 361-9208

Works to improve the education and increase the independence of individuals with severe disabilities. Holds annual conference. Quarterly "Journal of the Association for Persons with Severe Handicaps" and "TASH Newsletter" (both included with membership).

Technical Assistance for Special Populations Program (TASPP)
1310 South Sixth Street
Champaign, IL 61820
(217) 333-0807   FAX (217)244-5632

Provides resource and referral services to professionals working with individuals with special needs at secondary and postsecondary levels. Publishes "BRIEFS," which highlight critical vocational education issues and newsletter, "TASPP Bulletin;" offers information searches on a computerized database, all FREE.

Technical Assistance to Parent Programs (TAPP) Network
Federation for Children with Special Needs
95 Berkeley Street, Suite 104
Boston, MA 02116
(617) 482-2915 (V/TT)   In MA, (800) 331-0688

Provides technical assistance on health issues through parent training and information activities. Newsletter, "Coalition Quarterly," FREE.

PROFESSIONAL PUBLICATIONS

Ammerman, Robert T., Vincent B. Van Hasselt, and Michael Hersen
1991 "Parent-Child Problem-Solving Interactions in Families of Visually Impaired Youth" Journal of Pediatric Psychology 16(1):87-101

Barraga, Natalie C. and Jane N. Erin
1992 Visual Handicaps and Learning Austin, TX: Pro-Ed

Batshaw, Mark L.
1991 Your Child has A Disability Boston, MA: Little Brown

Chapman, Elizabeth K. and Juliet M. Stone
1988 The Visually Handicapped Child in Your Classroom Baltimore, MD: Brookes Publishing

Faye, Eleanor E., W. V. Padula, J. B. Padula, J. E. Gurland, M. L. Greenberg, and C. M. Hood
1984 "The Low Vision Child" pp. 437-475 in Eleanor E. Faye (ed.) Clinical Low Vision Boston, MA: Little Brown and Company

Gerry, Martin
1987 "Procedural Safeguards Insuring that Handicapped Children Receive a Free Appropriate Public Education" News Digest National Information Center for Children and Youth with Disabilities, PO Box 1492, Washington, D.C. 20013

Gill, Carol J.
1991 "Treating Families Coping with a Disability" Western Journal of Medicine 154(May):624-25

Gimblett, Roberta
1992 Peer Mentoring: A Support Group Model for College Students with Disabilities Association on Higher Education and Disability, PO Box 21192, Columbus, OH 43221-0192

Gobele, John L.
1984 Visual Disorders in the Handicapped Child New York, NY: Marcel Dekker

Goldie, D., S. Gormezano, and P. Raznik
1986 "Comprehensive Low Vision Services for Visually Impaired Children: A Function of Special Education" Journal of Visual Impairment and Blindness 80:844-848

Hebbeler, Kathleen, M., Barbara J. Smith, and Talbot L. Black
1991 "Federal Early Childhood Special Education Policy: A Model for the Improvement of Services for Children with Disabilities" Exceptional Children October/November, 104-112

Hritcko, Terese
1983 "Assessment of Children with Low Vision" pp. 105-137 in Randall T. Jose (ed.) Understanding Low Vision New York, NY: American Foundation for the Blind

Jan, James E., Ann M. Sykanda, and Maryke Groenveld
1990 "Habilitation and Rehabilitation of Visually Impaired and Blind Children" Pediatrician 17(3):202-207

Lagrow, Steve and Susan Vlahas Ponchillia
1989 "Children with Visual Impairments" pp. 133-186 in Anthony F. Rotatori and Robert A. Fox (eds.) Understanding Individuals with Low Incidence Handicaps Springfield, IL: Charles C. Thomas

National Information Center for Children and Youth with Disabilities
1987 Transition -- The Roles of Parents, Students, and Professionals National Information Center for Children and Youth with Disabilities, PO Box 1492, Washington, D.C. 20013

Orlansky, Michael
1988 "Assessment of Visually Impaired Infants and Preschool Children" pp. 93-107 in Theodore D. Wachs and Robert Sheehan (eds.) Assessment of Young Developmentally Disabled Children New York, NY: Plenum Press

Pogrund, Rona L., Diane L. Fazzi, and Jessical S. Lampert
1992 Early Focus: Working with Young Blind and Visually Impaired Children and Their Families New York, NY: American Foundation for the Blind

Rogow, Sally M.
1988 Helping the Visually Impaired Child with Developmental Problems New York, NY: Teachers College Press

Services for Independent Living
    With Feeling (curriculum for professionals working with parents of a child with a disability) Services for Independent Living, 25100 Euclid Avenue, Cleveland, OH 44117

Sisson, Lori, A. and Thomas J. Babeo
1992 "School-to-Work Transition of Students with Blindness or Visual Impairment" Journal of Vocational Rehabilitation 2(1):56-65

Spaulding, A.
1986 "Young People's Books Concerning Visual Impairment" Journal of Visual Impairment and Blindness 80:101-1018

Stotland, Judith
1984 "Relationship of Parents to Professionals: A Challenge to Professionals" Journal of Visual Impairment and Blindness 78:69-74

Texas School for the Blind
1991 Independent Living: A Curriculum with Adaptations for Students with Visual Impairments Texas School for the Blind, Business Office, 1100 West 45th Street, Austin, TX 78756-3494

Van Hasselt, Vincent B. and Lori A. Sisson
1987 "Visual Impairment" pp. 593-618 in Cynthia L. Frame and Johnny L. Matson (eds.) Handbook of Assessment in Childhood Psychopathology

Warnke, James W.
1991 "The Role of the Family in the Adjustment to Blindness or Visual Impairment" pp. 37-45 in Susan L. Greenblatt (ed.) Meeting the Needs of People with Vision Loss: A Multidisciplinary Perspective Lexington, MA: Resources for Rehabilitation
1991 "Special Needs of Children and Adolescents" pp. 61-69 in Susan L. Greenblatt (ed.) Meeting the Needs of People with Vision Loss: A Multidisciplinary Perspective Lexington, MA: Resources for Rehabilitation

Organizations

(In the listings below, telephone numbers have symbols V for voice and TT for text telephone where organizations have published this information.)

American Council of the Blind (ACB)
1155 15th Street, NW, Suite 720
Washington, DC 20005
(800) 424-8666   (202) 467-5081   FAX (202) 467-5085

National membership organization. Shares parenting information between blind/sighted parents of blind/sighted children. Also has a student division with chapters in many states. Makes referrals to local affiliates.

Beach Center on Families and Disability
c/o Institute for Life Span Studies
3111 Haworth Hall
Lawrence, KS 66045
(913) 864-7600   FAX (913) 864-7605

A federally funded center that conducts research and training related to families with members who have disabilities. Publications catalogue describes monographs and tapes related to family coping, professional roles, and service delivery, FREE. Publishes newsletter, "Families and Disability," FREE.

Canadian National Institute for the Blind (CNIB)
1931 Bayview Avenue
Toronto, Ontario M4G 4C8 Canada
(416) 480-7580   FAX (416) 480-7677

Provides counseling, life skills training, sight enhancement services, summer youth programs, teen and parent support groups, library services, and career development programs. Services vary from office to office (See "Appendix B: Division Offices of the Canadian National Institute for the Blind").

Clearinghouse on Disability Information
Office of Special Education and Rehabilitative Services (OSERS)
U.S. Department of Education
Room 3132 Switzer Building
Washington, DC 20202-2524
(202) 205-8723

Answers questions about services and programs for individuals of all ages with disabilities. Produces a variety of publications including newsletter, "OSERS in Print," which focuses on federal activities. FREE

Hadley School for the Blind
700 Elm Street
Winnetka, IL 60093
(800) 323-4238   In IL, (708) 446-8111

Offers correspondence courses for parents of children who are visually impaired or blind, FREE. Course catalogue available in LARGE PRINT, audiocassette, and braille. FREE

HEATH Resource Center
One Dupont Circle
Washington, DC 20036-1193
(800) 544-3284 (V/TT)   (202) 939-9320 (V/TT)   FAX (202) 833-4760

Provides information about the transition from high school to postsecondary education. Publishes newsletter, "Information from HEATH." Publishes "Students Who are Blind or Visually Impaired in Postsecondary Education," "Career Planning and Placement Strategies for Postsecondary Students with Disabilities," "How to Choose a College: Guide for the Student with a Disability" and "Vocational Rehabilitation Services: A Postsecondary Student Consumer's Guide." Publications list and all HEATH publications are FREE in standard print and audiocassette, or send a blank 3 1/2" or 5 1/4" double sided, double density disk and indicate choice of MS-DOS compatible or Macintosh.

Kids on the Block
9385-C Gerwig Lane
Columbia, MD 21046
(800) 368-5437   (410) 290-9095   FAX (410) 290-9358

A program that uses puppets to help students understand disabilities and chronic conditions. Various programs available, including blindness, diabetes, and sibling of a disabled child. Also publishes "The Kids on the Block" series of books, written for children in grades two to five, which feature children with chronic conditions or disabilities. "Business is Looking Up" is the story of a youngster with visual impairment who starts a small business. Question and answer sections about the characters' disabilities in each book. $12.95.

Learning Pillows
PO Box 631, New Town Branch
Boston, MA 02258
(617) 926-6974

A series of puppets and pillows, including Mr. Bug, Bumpedy Bumps, and the King and His Closet, that help young children with eye-hand coordination, visual discrimination, buttoning, and zipping, etc. Some pillows have coordinated stories on audiocassette and a parent/teacher activity guide. Prices range from $8.00 for puppets to $30.00 for pillows and audiocassettes plus shipping and handling.

National Alliance of Blind Students
c/o American Council of the Blind (ACB)
1155 15th Street, NW, Suite 720
Washington, DC 20005
(800) 424-8666   (202) 467-5081   FAX (202) 467-5085

Consumer group for students who are visually impaired or blind. Publishes "The Student Advocate," three times per year, in LARGE PRINT and audiocassette. Membership, $5.00.

National Association for Parents of Visually Impaired (NAPVI)
PO Box 317
Watertown, MA 02272-0317
(800) 562-6265

Promotes development of parent groups; provides information through conferences, publications, and quarterly newsletter, "Awareness." Local chapters in some states. FREE information packet. Membership, $20.00.

National Association for Visually Handicapped (NAVH)
22 West 21st Street
New York, NY 10010
(212) 889-3141

Sells and lends LARGE PRINT books for children. LARGE PRINT newsletter for youth,"In Focus," FREE

National Center for Youth with Disabilities (NCYD)
University of Minnesota
Box 721 UMHC
Harvard Street at East River Road
Minneapolis, MN 55455
(800) 333-6293   (612) 626-2825   (612) 624-3939 (TT)
FAX (612) 626-2134

An information center on adolescents with chronic illness and disabilities that provides access to research findings, resources, and advocacy for professional service providers and for parents. Maintains a national resource database and library with abstracts of current literature on disability and chronic illness; information about innovative programs; and a network of consultants who provide technical assistance. Publishes newsletter, "Connections," FREE.

National Federation of the Blind (NFB)
1800 Johnson Street
Baltimore, MD 21230
(410) 659-9314   FAX (410) 685-5653

The Parents of Blind Children Division sponsors seminars and workshops and provides information and support. Publishes "Future Reflections," a quarterly magazine with resources and guidelines, available in standard print and audiocassette. Membership, $8.00. FREE Parents Information Pack. Also produces two books on education of blind children: "Your School Includes a Blind Student," $3.75, and "A Resource Guide for Parents and Educators of Blind Children," $5.95. NFB's Student Division provides support to students through chapters in many states.

National Information Center for Children and Youth with Disabilities (NICHCY)
PO Box 1492
Washington, DC 20013-1492
(800) 999-5599   (703) 893-8614 (TT)

A federally funded clearinghouse that provides information about disabilities and referral guides. Publishes newsletter, "News Digest," which focuses on special topics such as "Assistive Technology," "Children with Handicaps, Parent and Family Issues," and "Understanding Sibling Issues." FREE

National Library Service for the Blind and Physically Handicapped (NLS)
1291 Taylor Street, NW
Washington, DC 20542
(800) 424-8567 or 8572 (Reference Section)
(800) 424-9100 (to receive application)
(202) 707-5100   FAX (202) 707-0712

Provides talking book equipment on loan and recorded and braille books for preschoolers, students, and adults through a network of regional libraries. Publishes "Parents' Guide to the Development of Pre-School Handicapped Children: Resources and Services," "Selected Readings for Parents of Preschool Handicapped Children," and "From School to Working Life: Resources and Services," standard print. FREE.

National Resume Database for Students With Disabilities
Association on Higher Education and Disability (AHEAD)
PO Box 21192
Columbus, OH 43221-0192
(614) 488-4972 (V/TT)   FAX (614) 488-1174

A database that enables students with disabilities to disseminate their resumes to potential employers. The employer receives information about the students' qualifications, not their disabilities. It is up to the student and employer to discuss accommodations. Students may obtain a database form by sending a self-addressed, stamped envelope to AHEAD. Forms may also be available in disabled student service offices on campus. No charge for students. Employers interested in purchasing or searching the database should contact Resume Link, PO Box 218, Hilliard, OH 43026 (614) 771-7087

PACER Center (Parent Advocacy Coalition for Educational Rights)
4826 Chicago Avenue South
Minneapolis, MN 55417-1098
(612) 827-2966 (V/TT)   In MN, (800) 537-2237   FAX (612) 827-3065

A coalition of disability organizations which offers information about laws, procedures, parents' rights and responsibilities. Publishes the "Pacesetter," three times per year, FREE; the "Advocate," six times per year, $12.00; "Early Childhood Connection," for parents of young children with disabilities, three times per year, FREE; and "Computer Monitor," which describes computers and software for children with disabilities, three times per year, FREE. FREE catalogue.

Parent Education and Assistance for Kids (PEAK)
6055 Lehman Drive, Suite 101
Colorado Springs, CO 80918
(800) 284-0251   (719) 531-9400   (719) 531-9403 (V/TT)
FAX (719) 531-9452

A center that promotes the integration of children with disabilities in the regular classroom. Provides referrals for parents and technical assistance to school systems. Publishes newsletter, "Speak Out" (in English and Spanish), $9.00 for out of state professionals; FREE for others.

Pediatric Projects, Inc.
PO Box 571555
Tarzana, CA 91357
(800) 947-0947   (818) 705-3660   FAX (818) 705-3660

Produces toys and books that help children understand visual impairment and other disabilities. Prices range from $12.95 to $59.95. Publishes "Medical Toys & Books," a guide to toys and books for children and adolescents with disabilities and chronic conditions. Subscription, $14.00. "Vision, Vision Impairment, & Blindness," ($2.00) and "Siblings of Disabled or Ill Children," ($8.00) are two bibliographies of references for children with disabilities.

American Printing House for the Blind (APH)
1839 Frankfort Avenue
Louisville, KY 40206-0085
(800) 223-1839   (502) 895-2405   FAX (502) 895-1509

Sells infant, preschool, kindergarten, primary, and multihandicapped aids including games, teaching aids, and texts. Titles include "Beginnings--A Practical Guide for Parents and Teachers of Visually Impaired Babies," $7.50; "Hands On: Functional Activities for Visually Impaired Preschoolers," kit, $132.93, guidebook, $11.45; "Parents and Visually Impaired Infants," $26.00, and a videotape, "Playing the Crucial Role in Your Child's Development," $20.00. Request a preschool packet. Also publishes "Century Series Braille Books."

Blind Childrens Center
4120 Marathon Street
PO Box 29159
Los Angeles, CA 90029-0159
(800) 222-3566   In CA, (800) 222-3567   (213) 664-2153
FAX (213) 665-3828

Provides resources and support to parents. Publications include "First Steps: A Handbook for Teaching Young Children Who Are Visually Impaired," $19.95 plus $3.99 shipping and handling; "Talk to Me I," "Talk to Me II," "Heart-to-Heart - Parents of Blind and Partially Sighted Children Talk About Their Feelings," "Move with Me," and "Learning to Play: Common Concerns for the Visually Impaired Preschool Child," all available in English and Spanish at $1.50 each; "Dancing Cheek to Cheek," English only, $3.00; and "Reaching, Crawling, Walking: Let's Get Moving," $3.00, available in English and Spanish. Add 20% for postage.

Bolinda Press
PO Box 14402
Shawnee Mission, KS 66285
(800) 848-8810   FAX (913) 894-5526

Hardcover and paperback titles for adults and children. FREE catalogue.

BOOMERANG!
123 Townsend, Suite 636
San Francisco, CA 94107
(800) 333-7858

Monthly current events magazine for children on standard audiocassette. $39.95 for 12 issues; $12.95 for a three month trial subscription; $5.95 for a single issue.

Building Integration With the I.E.P.
by Barbara E. Buswell and Judy Veneris
Parent Education and Assistance for Kids (PEAK)
6055 Lehman Drive, Suite 101
Colorado Springs, CO 80918
(800) 284-0251   (719) 531-9400   (719) 531-9403 (V/TT)
FAX (719) 531-9452

A booklet that helps parents understand what they can do and expect from the I.E.P. meetings. $5.00

Can Do Video Series
Visually Impaired Preschool Services
1215 South Third Street
Louisville, KY 40203
(502) 636-3207

A series of five videotapes that depict six families with children who are visually impaired, ranging from 14 months to six years. Write for description of tapes. Each tape may be purchased separately for $39.95 or the entire set may be purchased for $179.95. $10.00 shipping charge for up to five tapes.

Children's Braille Book Club
National Braille Press (NBP)
88 St. Stephen Street
Boston, MA 02115
(617) 266-6160   FAX (617) 437-0456

Braille pages are inserted into standard print children's books. FREE membership provides monthly notices with no obligation to buy; $100.00 annual subscription automatically provides one print-braille book per month.

Cornerstone Large Print Books
Bantam Doubleday Delacorte Library Services
100 Pine Avenue, Dept. CDM 1
Holmes, PA 19043
(800) 345-8112

Catalogue of LARGE PRINT books for children and adolescents. FREE

Directory of College Facilities and Services for People with Disabilities, third edition
Oryx Press, Phoenix, AZ
(800) 279-6799   FAX (800) 279-4663

Describes the physical facilities, special services, and academic programs for colleges throughout the U.S. and Canada. $115.00

The Exceptional Parent
PO Box 3000, Dept. EP
Denville, NJ 07834
(800) 247-8080

This magazine emphasizes problem solving and provides practical information about raising and educating a child with a disability. Eight issues per year. Subscription for individuals, $18.00; schools, libraries, and agencies, $24.00

Getting in Touch with Play: Creative Play Environments for Children with Visual Impairments
Lighthouse National Center for Vision and Child Development (NCVCD)
800 Second Avenue
New York, NY 10017
(800) 334-5497 (V/TT)   (212) 808-0077   FAX (212) 808-0110

A book that includes a set of diagrams and photographs of playground settings that encourage children with visual impairments to play. $8.00

Individualized Education Programs (Reprint 2/90)
National Information Center for Children and Youth with Disabilities (NICHCY)
PO Box 1492
Washington, DC 20013
(800) 999-5599 (V/TT)   In Washington, DC area, (703) 893-6061 (V/TT)

This publication describes the purposes and contents of the IEP, the responsibility of the state education agency, the role of parents, and the requirements for holding meetings. FREE

Just Enough to Know Better
by Eileen Curran
National Braille Press (NBP)
88 St. Stephen Street
Boston, MA 02115
(617) 266-6160   FAX (617) 437-0456

This self-paced workbook teaches beginning braille skills to sighted parents. $12.50

LARGE PRINT Books for Young Readers
G.K. Hall
Order Dept.
100 Front Street, Box 500
Riverside, NJ 08075-7500
(800) 257-5755

FREE catalogue of LARGE PRINT books for children and adolescents.

Lifeprints
Blindskills, Inc.
Box 5181
Salem, OR 97304
(503) 581-4224

Magazine with focus on careers and life skills of youth and adults who are visually impaired or blind. LARGE PRINT, audiocassette, and braille subscriptions, $15.00. Sample copy, $3.00

Mom Can't See Me
by Sally Hobart Alexander
Macmillan Publishing Company
100 Front Street, Box 500
Riverside, NJ 08075-7500
(800) 257-5755   (609) 461-6500

Written from her nine year old daughter's point of view, the author describes family life with a mother who is blind. LARGE PRINT. $14.95

Opening Doors: Strategies for Including All Students in Regular Education
by C. Beth Schaffner and Barbara E. Buswell
Parent Education and Assistance for Kids (PEAK)
6055 Lehman Drive, Suite 101
Colorado Springs, CO 80918
(800) 284-0251   (719) 531-9400   (719) 531-9403 (V/TT)
FAX (719) 531-9452

Written for educators and parents, this book contains practical information about integrating students with disabilities into regular classrooms. $10.00

An Orientation and Mobility Primer for Families and Young Children
by B. Dodson-Burk and E. W. Hill
American Foundation for the Blind (AFB)
15 West 16th Street
New York, NY 10011
(800) 232-5463   (212) 620-2000

Provides information about orientation and mobility training. $8.95 plus $3.00 shipping and handling.

Pathways to Independence: Orientation and Mobility Skills for Your Infant and Toddler
Lighthouse National Center for Vision and Child Development
800 Second Avenue
New York, NY 10017
(800) 334-5497 (V/TT)   (212) 808-0077   FAX (212) 808-0110

Discusses basic orientation and mobility skills and suggests games and activities for the child with vision loss. $2.50

Questions Kids Ask About Blindness
National Federation of the Blind (NFB)
1800 Johnson Street
Baltimore, MD 21230
(410) 659-9314   FAX (410) 685-5653

Answers general questions about blindness, braille, canes, guide dogs, and the abilities of individuals who are visually impaired or blind. Describes a typical day in the life of a blind sixth grader attending public school. $3.50

Seedlings
PO Box 2395
Livonia, MI 48151-0395
(313) 427-8552

Publishes inexpensive children's storybooks in braille. FREE catalogue.

Since Owen
by Charles R. Callanan
Johns Hopkins University Press, Baltimore, MD

Written by the father of a child with a disability, this book describes the experience of obtaining an appropriate education and finding resources. $16.95

The Student with Albinism in the Regular Classroom
by Julia Robertson Ashley
National Organization for Albinism and Hypopigmentation (NOAH)
1500 Locust Street, Suite 1816
Philadelphia, PA 19102
(800) 473-2310   (215) 545-2322

Describes special needs of children with albinism and suggests adaptations for classroom and nonclassroom activities. LARGE PRINT. $3.50

They Don't Come with Manuals
Fanlight Productions
47 Halifax Street
Boston, MA 02130
(617) 524-0980   FAX (617) 524-8838

A videotape in which parents talk about their own experiences raising a child with a disability. 29 minutes. Rental: $50.00 a day; $100.00 a week. Purchase: $195.00

Travel Tales - A Mobility Storybook
Mostly Mobility
7100 Route 183
Bethel, PA 19507

Designed to teach mobility to children in preschool through third grade, this book may be used by parents of children who are visually impaired or blind, classroom teachers, special education teachers, as well as orientation and mobility teachers. $22.00

Vision in Children - Normal and Abnormal
by Dr. Lea Hyvarinen
Canadian Deaf-Blind and Rubella Association
747 2nd Avenue East, Suite 4
Owen Sound, Ontario N4K 2G9 Canada
(519) 372-1333 (V/TT)   FAX (519) 372-1334

Compares visual development of children with normal vision and those with visual impairments; discusses the special needs of children with multiple disabilities; and recommends play and games for early motor development. Available in English and French. $7.00 (plus $2.50 for shipping outside Canada) Canadian funds.

Financial aid for students with disabilities is provided by the U.S. Department of Education and administered by state departments of vocational rehabilitation. Each state has its own eligibility criteria. Contact your state agency for more information (See "Appendix A: State Agencies for Individuals Who Are Visually Impaired or Blind").

The following organizations offer academic scholarships. Special qualification criteria are noted when applicable.

American Council of the Blind (ACB)
1155 15th Street, NW, Suite 720
Washington, DC 20005
(800) 424-8666   (202) 467-5081   FAX (202) 467-5085

American Foundation for the Blind (AFB)
15 West 16th Street
New York, NY 10011
(800) 232-5463   (212) 620-2000

Association for Education and Rehabilitation of the Blind and Visually Impaired (AER)
206 North Washington Street, Suite 320
Alexandria, VA 22314
(703) 548-1884

Administers scholarships for postsecondary students preparing for a career serving individuals who are visually impaired or blind. The Ferrell Scholarship requires that applicants be legally blind. The Telesensory Scholarship requires that applicants be current members of AER. Applications deadline of April 15 in even numbered years.

Christian Record Services
4444 South 52nd Street
Lincoln, NE 68506
(402) 488-0981

Provides financial assistance to students who are legally blind and who are planning to attend an undergraduate college. Applications must be received by April 1 for the following academic year.

Council of Citizens with Low Vision International (CCLVI)
5707 Brockton Drive, #302
Indianapolis, IN 46220-5481
(800) 733-2258   (317) 254-1185   FAX (317) 251-6588

Awards the CCLVI-Telesensory Scholarship of $1,000.00 to an undergraduate student who has low vision but is not totally blind. Application deadline of April 1. The Carl E. Foley Scholarship awards $1,000.00 to a graduate student studying vision rehabilitation at one of four designated institutions.

Dominican College of San Rafael
Ted Blair, Chair, Department of Music
50 Acacia Avenue
San Rafael, CA 94901-8008
(415) 485-3275

Awards the Rho Barrett Music Scholarship to a student who is legally blind and a music major.

Fordham University
c/o Amy Reiss
Morrison, Cohen, Singer, and Weinstein
750 Lexington Avenue
New York, NY 10022
(212) 535-4764

Provides scholarships for law students who are blind.

Foundation for Science and the Handicapped
Rebecca F. Smith
115 South Brainard Avenue
La Grange, IL 60525

Awards a $1,000.00 scholarship to students entering or continuing in a Master's degree program in mathematics, science, medicine, engineering, or computer science. Annual application deadline is December 1.

George Washington University
Disabled Student Services
Rice Hall, Room 401
2121 Eye Street, NW
Washington, DC 20052

Provides financial assistance to part-time students who are visually impaired or blind through the Barbara Jackman Zuckert Scholarship. Applications must be postmarked by May 30.

National Federation of the Blind (NFB)
Attn: Peggy Pinder
814 4th Avenue, Suite 200
Grinnell, IA 50112
(515) 236-2147

Recording for the Blind (RFB)
20 Roszel Road
Princeton, NJ 08540
(800) 221-4792   In NJ, (609) 452-0606   FAX (609) 987-8116

Scholastic achievement awards for legally blind college students.

The Federal Educational and Scholarship Funding Guide
Grayco Publishing
PO Box 1291
West Warwick, RI 02893

Lists more than 125 organizations that make grants in all aspects of education. $39.95

Federal Student Aid
Federal Student Aid Center
PO Box 84
Washington, DC 20044

This audiocassette describes financial aid available to students with disabilities, including visual impairment; includes federal grant, loan, and work-study programs; scholarships; and discusses the rights of students with disabilities. FREE

Financial Aid for Students with Disabilities
HEATH Resource Center
One Dupont Circle
Washington, DC 20036-1193
(800) 544-3284   (202) 939-9320 (V/TT)   FAX (202) 833-4760

Covers the various types of financial aid, such as grants, loans, and work; describes vocational rehabilitation services; and lists organizations which provide scholarships as well as resource directories. Standard print and audiocassette, or send a blank 3 1/2" or 5 1/4" double sided, double density disk and indicate choice of MS-DOS compatible or Macintosh. FREE

Financial Aid from the U.S. Department of Education: The Student Guide
Office of Student Financial Assistance
Office of Postsecondary Education
U.S. Department of Education
400 Maryland Avenue, SW
Washington, DC 20202

A booklet describing the various scholarship, loan, and work-study programs funded by the Department of Education. FREE

ELDERS

In 1989, individuals age 65 and over accounted for 12% of the American population; this proportion is projected to increase rapidly as the baby boom generation enters its later years. Since visual impairment is most prevalent among the older population, it is also projected that the number of people with visual impairments will increase substantially. Currently, over eight percent of the population age 65 and over have visual impairments; for the age group 75 and over the proportion increases to over ten percent (U.S. Department of Health and Human Services: 1991).

The major causes of vision loss among elders are macular degeneration, cataract, diabetic retinopathy, and glaucoma. Individuals over age 65 are at ten times greater risk for legal blindness than younger people (Pizzarello: 1987). The rate of visual impairment and blindness is higher for institutionalized elders than for non-institutionalized elders. Whitmore (1989) found that 30% of the residents he examined in a nursing home were legally blind.

Most elders live in the community, and nearly one-third (30.5%) live alone (U.S. Department of Health and Human Services: 1991). Only 5% live in nursing homes (Fowles: 1991). A study of elders living in the community (Branch et al.: 1989) found that elders with vision loss represent a population of "extensive unmet needs." This study found that elders with vision loss had difficulty carrying out the tasks of everyday living required to continue living in the community, but they did not receive adequate social services, health services, or mental health services. According to Branch and his colleagues, neither the aging service network nor the blindness system has addressed the needs of elders with vision loss adequately. A study by Stuen (1991) found that staff in 83% of the responding aging agencies felt they needed more information about visual impairment.

Duffy and Beliveau-Tobey (1991) observed that the high prevalence of vision loss among residents of long term care facilities has been recognized by many experts, yet little has been done to train the staff at these facilities to cope with the problem. Their national survey and test of a pilot in-service curriculum suggest that training the staff of long term care facilities can help alleviate many of the residents' problems that are associated with visual impairment.

Along with the problem of vision loss, many elders have other special needs. Stroke, arthritis, hearing loss, and heart conditions pose additional challenges for medical and rehabilitation professionals who work with elders with vision loss. A team approach to medical/rehabilitation treatment plans is essential, especially when multiple conditions are involved. Medications for hypertension or allergies may affect a patient's eye condition; lack of response to a hearing assessment might be attributable to central vision loss; and vision loss due to stroke may sometimes be misinterpreted as mental confusion.

Rehabilitation services for people who are visually impaired or blind were originally designed for children and employable adults, since the goal of rehabilitation was to enable these individuals to work or to return to work. In recent years, rehabilitation services have been expanded to include elders, and the role of "homemaker" is considered a justifiable rehabilitation goal. According to Crews et al. (1987) many agencies are extending traditional services to this "new" population through "independent living programs;" skills training (rehabilitation teaching, orientation and mobility skills); counseling; and information and referral services. Nearly half the states that offer independent living programs to elders also include low vision services, advocacy or self/advocacy, peer counseling, and housing assistance.

Both public and private organizations as well as self-help groups are available to help elders with vision loss in most major metropolitan areas. The state agency that serves individuals who are visually impaired or blind is a good source of information about services. Many state agencies provide special services to elders with vision loss under the federally funded program, Independent Living Services for Older Blind Individuals, authorized by Title VII, Part C of the Rehabilitation Act as amended. Senior centers, home health care providers, and special services for elders located at hospitals should all be able to accommodate the special needs of elders with vision loss and other disabilities.

References

Branch, Lawrence G., Amy Horowitz, and Cheryl Carr
1989 "The Implications for Everyday Life of Incident Self-Reported Visual Decline Among People over Age 65 Living in the Community" The Gerontologist 29:359-365

Crews, J.E., W.D. Frey, and P.E. Peterson
1987 "Independent Living for the Handicapped Elderly Community: A National View" Journal of Visual Impairment and Blindness 81(September):305-308

Duffy, Maureen and Monica Beliveau-Tobey
1991 "Providing Services to Visually Impaired Elders in Long Term Care Facilities: A Multidisciplinary Approach" pp. 93-107 in Susan L. Greenblatt (ed.) Meeting the Needs of People with Vision Loss: A Multidisciplinary Perspective Lexington, MA: Resources for Rehabilitation

Fowles, Donald G.
1991 A Profile of Older Americans 1991 Washington, DC: American Association of Retired Persons

Pizzarello, Louis D.
1987 "The Dimensions of the Problem of Eye Disease Among the Elderly" Ophthalmology 94:9:1191

Stuen, Cynthia
1991 "Awareness of Resources for Visually Impaired Older Adults among the Aging Network"
Journal of Gerontological Social Work 17(3/4):165-179

U.S. Bureau of the Census
1986 Disability, Functional Limitation, and Health Insurance Coverage: 1984-85 Current
Population Reports, Series P-70, No. 8, U.S. Government Printing Office, Washington,
DC

U.S. Department of Health and Human Services
1991 Aging in America: Trends and Projections Washington, D.C.: U.S. Department of
Health and Human Services DHHS Publication No. (FCoA) 91-28001

Whitmore, Wayne G.
1989 "Eye Disease in a Geriatric Nursing Home Population" Ophthalmology 96:393-398

Amanda McNeil: Living Independently with Vision Loss

Amanda MacNeil is a 77 year old widow who has age-related macular degeneration. She lives alone in her own home and is a participant at the senior center.

The activities director at the senior center, Carla Shapiro, has recently noticed that Mrs. MacNeil appears to be losing weight, is not dressing as carefully as she used to, and is hesitant in moving around the center. When Ms Shapiro asked Mrs. MacNeil if she was having any health problems, Mrs. MacNeil responded that she "just isn't interested in food much anymore." Several additional questions revealed that Mrs. MacNeil has become very apprehensive about cooking since she had burned herself several times. When Ms Shapiro asked Mrs. MacNeil about her vision problems, Mrs. MacNeil responded that she no longer visits the ophthalmologist, because he said nothing could be done to improve her vision.

Ms Shapiro had previously contracted with the team of Dr. Sheila Burns, an ophthalmologist, and Dr. Harvey Belmont, an optometrist, to conduct vision screenings at the senior center. She asked Mrs. MacNeil if she would consider setting up an appointment with these service providers. Mrs. MacNeil agreed, and an appointment was scheduled for the following week.

Dr. Burns examined Mrs. MacNeil and confirmed the diagnosis of age-related macular degeneration. With an acuity of 20/200 in each eye, Mrs. MacNeil is legally blind and eligible for state services. Dr. Burns explained to Mrs. MacNeil that she will be registered with the state commission for the blind. Mrs. MacNeil protested, fearing the term "legally blind," but Dr. Burns explained that this term entitles Mrs. MacNeil to government services and does not indicate that she will lose all useful vision. After hearing this explanation, Mrs. MacNeil ceased her protests and also accepted a referral for a low vision examination from Dr. Belmont.

Dr. Belmont's low vision evaluation resulted in the prescription of a telescope for reading signs on the bus, several magnifiers, and glare control glasses. He demonstrated a closed circuit television to Mrs. MacNeil, who was intrigued, but

Continued on next page

134

she decided to wait for her visit from the state agency worker prior to making any purchases. Dr. Belmont informed her that services from a rehabilitation teacher can improve her cooking skills and help with her other activities.

The rehabilitation teacher from the state agency, Jeffrey Booth, visited on a weekly basis, practicing cooking with Mrs. MacNeil in her own kitchen. Mr. Booth marked the stove's temperature controls with a tactile substance as a guide to various settings and recommended a flame-tamer device set over a burner in order to prevent burns. He suggested purchasing a small microwave oven for safely heating leftovers, boiling water, and cooking simple dishes such as baked potatoes and microwave-ready meals.

Mr. Booth also showed Mrs. MacNeil how to move more safely around her apartment using tactile cues and setting up simple systems to avoid accidents, such as marking her steps with bright colored tape, placing a safety rail and non-skid mat on the tub, and replacing the light bulbs with higher watt bulbs. He also suggested nightlights in the bathroom, the hall, and in various other sites. Mr. Booth and Mrs. MacNeil reorganized her clothing, hanging matching outfits together and using plastic storage boxes to help her find items more easily.

Following several months of lessons from Mr. Booth, Mrs. MacNeil has gained weight and is once again an active participant at the senior center. When she discussed her progress with the others at the senior center, many were surprised to learn that it is possible to continue living as independently as Mrs. MacNeil does, in spite of her vision loss. They asked Ms Shapiro if she would schedule a program so Mr. Booth can discuss the services he provides through the state agency that serves individuals who are visually impaired or blind.

(In the listings below, telephone numbers have symbols V for voice and TT for text telephone where organizations have published this information.)

American Geriatrics Society (AGS)
770 Lexington Avenue, Suite 300
New York, NY 10021
(212) 308-1414

Membership organization of physicians and other health care professionals. Sponsors an annual meeting and continuing medical education courses. Publishes "Journal of the American Geriatrics Society" and "Senior Medical Review."

Gerontological Society of America (GSA)
1275 K Street, NW, Suite 350
Washington, DC 20005-4006
(202) 842-1275

National membership organization for researchers, educators, and professionals in the field of aging. Maintains the GSA Information Service, a computerized data base, listing experts in aging topics and issues and a calendar of conferences on aging. Holds annual scientific meetings. Publishes "The Gerontologist" and "The Journals of Gerontology," with sections on social sciences, biological sciences, medical sciences, and psychological sciences. Monthly newsletter, "Gerontology News."

Lighthouse National Center for Vision and Aging (NCVA)
800 Second Avenue
New York, NY 10017
(800) 334-5497 (V/TT)   (212) 808-0077   FAX (212) 808-0110

Provides information on vision problems faced by older people and how these problems can be treated. Sells community education materials. Newsletter, "Aging and Vision Loss," published three times a year, FREE.

National Institute on Aging (NIA)
National Institutes of Health
9000 Rockville Pike
Bethesda, MD 20205
(301) 496-1752

A federal agency that supports basic and clinical research on a broad range of issues that affect elders. Funds Geriatric Research and Training Centers. Information about Requests for Proposals and Requests for Applications is published in the "NIH Guide for Grants and

Contracts," published weekly, FREE. Available from NIH Office of Grants Inquiries, Division of Research Grants, Westwood Building, Room 449, Bethesda, MD 20892 (301) 496-7441. Professional and consumer information publications available. FREE publications list.

Research and Training Center on Aging
Rancho Los Amigos Medical Center
PO Box 3500
Downey, CA 90242
(213) 940-7402

A federally funded center that conducts research on geriatric rehabilitation and service delivery issues. Conducts conferences, develops curricula, and publishes a newsletter, "Geriatric Rehabilitation PREVIEW," FREE.

PROFESSIONAL PUBLICATIONS

Abramson, Marcia and Paula M. Lovas
1988 Aging and Sensory Change: An Annotated Bibliography The Gerontological Society of America, 1275 K Street, NW, Suite 350, Washington, DC 20005-4006

Ageline
A bibliographic database that provides citations and abstracts on social, psychological, and health issues related to aging. Custom searches available through professional libraries, through the Dialog Information Services, and BRS Information Technologies. Contact American Association of Retired Persons, 601 E Street, NW, Washington, DC 20049, for an information packet (FREE) and a "Thesaurus of Aging Terminology," $7.00.

Ainlay, Stephen C.
1989 Day Brought Back My Night: Aging and New Vision Loss New York, NY: Routledge
1988 "Aging and New Vision Loss: Disruptions of the Here and Now" Journal of Social Issues 44:79-94

Biegel, David E., Marcia K. Petchers, Arlene Snyder, and Beverly Beisgen
1989 "Unmet Needs and Barriers to Service Delivery for the Blind and Visually Impaired Elderly" The Gerontologist 29(1):86-91

Canadian National Institute for the Blind
1991 Optimizing the Independence of Blind and Visually Impaired Seniors Canadian National Institute for the Blind, Department of Rehabilitation, 1931 Bayview Avenue, Toronto, Ontario M464C8

Crews, John E.
1988 "No One Left to Push: The Public Policy of Aging and Blindness" Educational Gerontology 14:399-409

Deichman, Elizabeth S. and Regina Kociecki (eds.)
1989 Working with the Elderly: An Introduction Buffalo, NY: Prometheus Books

Di Stefano, Anthony F. and Sheree J. Aston
1986 "Rehabilitation for the Blind and Visually Impaired Elderly" pp. 203 -217 in Stanley J. Brody and George E. Ruff (eds.) Aging and Rehabilitation New York, NY: Springer Publishing Company

Duffy, Maureen and Monica Beliveau-Tobey
1992 New Independence for Older Persons with Vision Loss in Long-Term Care Facilities AWARE, PO Box 96, Mohegan Lake, NY 10547

Goodman, Harriet
1985 "Serving the Elderly Blind: A Generic Approach" Journal of Gerontological Social Work 8:153-168

Kosnik, William, Robert Sekuler, and Donald Kline
1990 "Self-Reported Visual Problems of Older Drivers" Human Factors 32(5):597-608

Kosnik, William, Laura Winslow, Donald Kline, Kenneth Rasinski, and Robert Sekuler
1988 "Visual Changes in Daily Life Throughout Adulthood" Journal of Gerontology 43:3:63-70

Myers, Jane E.
1983 "Rehabilitation Counseling for Older Disabled Persons: The State of the Art" Journal of Applied Rehabilitation Counseling 14:3:48-52

National Institute on Aging (NIA)
    NIA Research Bulletin Gaithersburg, MD: NIA Information Center

Orr, Alberta L.
1991 Vision and Aging: Crossroads for Service Delivery New York, NY: American Foundation for the Blind

Rosenbloom, Alfred A. and Meredith W. Morgan, (eds.)
1986 Vision and Aging: General and Clinical Perspectives Stoneham, MA: Butterworth

Weber, Nancy D.
1992 Vision and Aging Issues in Social Work Practice Binghamton, NY: Haworth Press (Also published as volume 17, #3/4 of the Journal of Gerontological Social Work, 1991)

138

REFERRAL RESOURCES

Organizations

(In the listings below, telephone numbers have symbols V for voice and TT for text telephone where organizations have published this information.)

<u>Lighthouse National Center for Vision and Aging</u> (NCVA)
800 Second Avenue
New York, NY 10017
(800) 334-5497 (V/TT)   (212) 808-0077   FAX (212) 808-0110

Promotes better understanding of vision; provides information on vision problems faced by older people and how these problems can be treated. Sells community education materials. FREE newsletter.

<u>National Institute on Aging</u> (NIA)
NIA Information Center
PO Box 8057
Gaithersburg, MD 20898-8057
(301) 495-3455

Clearinghouse for information on aging. Publishes LARGE PRINT fact sheet series, "Age Page," which focuses on issues faced by elders, including "Aging and Your Eyes." FREE

Aging and Vision Loss
Resources for Rehabilitation
33 Bedford Street, Suite 19A
Lexington, MA 02173
(617) 862-6455   FAX (617) 861-7517

Designed for distribution by professionals, this LARGE PRINT (18 point bold type) publication describes organizations and publications for elders with vision loss. Minimum purchase, 25 copies. $1.25 per copy plus shipping and handling. Discounts available for purchases of 100 or more copies. See order form on last page of this book.

Caring for the Visually Impaired Older Person
Minneapolis Society for the Blind
1936 Lyndale Avenue South
Minneapolis, MN 55403
(612) 871-2222 (V/TT, FAX)   In MN, (800) 843-0619

Intended as a guide for long-term care facility staff, this booklet offers many helpful suggestions for anyone facing vision loss. $10.00 plus $2.50 shipping and handling.

Coping with the Diagnosis of Sight Loss
Resources for Rehabilitation
33 Bedford Street, Suite 19A
Lexington, MA 02173
(617) 862-6455   FAX (617) 861-7517

An audiocassette in which three consumers, two of them over age 55, discuss their experiences with vision loss. $12.00 plus $3.00 shipping and handling.

Eighty-Eight Easy-To-Make Aids for Older People
by Don Caston
Hartley & Marks, Publishers
Box 147
Point Roberts, WA 98281
(206) 945-2017

Practical adaptations for the home with step-by-step instructions. $11.95, plus $1.50 postage and handling.

A Handbook for Senior Citizens: Rights, Resources and Responsibilities
by Ramona Walhof
National Federation of the Blind
1800 Johnson Street
Baltimore, MD 21230
(410) 659-9314   FAX (410) 685-5653

Practical advice for individuals with vision loss, their families, and professionals. $5.95

I Keep Five Pairs of Glasses in a Flower Pot
by Henrietta Levner
National Association for Visually Handicapped (NAVH)
22 West 21st Street
New York, NY 10010
(212) 889-3141

Describes an older woman's experience in learning to live with low vision caused by macular degeneration. LARGE PRINT. $2.00

Living with Age-Related Macular Degeneration
Resources for Rehabilitation
33 Bedford Street, Suite 19A
Lexington, MA 02173
(617) 862-6455   FAX (617) 861-7517

Designed for distribution by professionals, this LARGE PRINT publication describes service organizations and publications that help people with macular degeneration. Minimum purchase, 25 copies. $1.25 per copy. Discounts available for purchases of 100 or more copies. See order form on last page of book.

Living with Vision Loss: A Handbook for Caregivers
Canadian National Institute for the Blind (CNIB)
Rehabilitation Department
1931 Bayview Avenue
Toronto, Ontario M4G 4C8 Canada
(416) 480-7626   FAX (416) 480-7677

Practical suggestions for everyday living with visual impairment or blindness. Includes community and CNIB resources. $12.50, Canadian funds.

Look Out for Annie
Lighthouse National Center on Vision and Aging (NCVA)
800 Second Avenue
New York, NY 10017
(800) 334-5497 (V/TT)   (212) 808-0077   FAX (212) 808-0110

A videotape which portrays an elderly woman with macular degeneration and her interactions with family, friends, and other elders at the senior center. Discussion guide included. $35.00, VHS or BETA format.

Making Life More Livable
by Irving R. Dickman
American Foundation for the Blind
15 West 16th Street
New York, NY 10011
(800) 232-5463   (212) 620-2000   FAX (212) 727-7418

Offers simple adaptations to make the home safer for people with vision impairment. $12.95 plus $3.00 shipping and handling. Also available on four-track audiocassette on loan through regional branches of the National Library Service for the Blind and Physically Handicapped. RC 22319.

Out of the Corner of My Eye: Living with Vision Loss in Later Life
by Nicolette Pernod Ringgold
American Foundation for the Blind (AFB)
15 West 16th Street
New York, NY 10011
(800) 232-5463   (212) 620-2000   FAX (212) 620-2105

Written by a woman who became legally blind due to macular degeneration in her late 70's, this book offers practical advice and encouragement for elders with vision loss. LARGE PRINT and audiocassette, $14.95 plus $3.00 shipping and handling.

Resources for Elders with Disabilities
Resources for Rehabilitation
33 Bedford Street, Suite 19A
Lexington, MA 02173
(617) 862-6455   FAX (617) 861-7517

A LARGE PRINT resource directory that describes services and products that elders with disabilities need to function independently. Includes chapters on vision loss, hearing loss, arthritis, diabetes, osteoporosis, Parkinson's disease, falls, and stroke. Updated biennially. $39.95 plus $5.00 shipping and handling See order form on last page of this book.

Self-Help/Mutual Aid Support Groups for Visually Impaired Older Persons: A Guide and Directory
Lighthouse National Center for Vision and Aging (NCVA)
800 Second Avenue
New York, NY 10017
(800) 334-5497 (V/TT)   (212) 808-0077   FAX (212) 808-0110

Lists local support groups throughout the U.S. $10.00

Self-Help Publications for Visually Impaired Individuals and Professionals
VISIONS
817 Broadway, 11th floor
New York, NY 10003
(212) 477-3800   FAX (212) 477-6613

Home study kits for self-help rehabilitation with audiocassettes, LARGE PRINT transcript, and performance evaluation criteria. Instructor manuals also available. Courses include Basic Indoor Mobility, Housekeeping Skills, Personal Management, and Sensory Development. HINTS booklets, "Ideas," available in English and Spanish, and "Getting Around Your Home," provide information for individuals and their families; $3.00 each. FREE catalogue.

Talking Books for Seniors
National Library Service for the Blind and Physically Handicapped (NLS)
1291 Taylor Street, NW
Washington, DC 20542
(800) 424-8567 or 8572 (Reference Section)
(800) 424-9100 (to receive application)
(202) 707-5100   FAX (202) 707-0712

This brochure promotes the use of talking books by seniors and describes how to receive them.

Work Sight
Lighthouse National Center on Vision and Aging (NCVA)
800 Second Avenue
New York, NY 10017
(800) 334-5497 (V/TT)   (212) 808-0077   FAX (212) 808-0110

This videotape discusses age-related vision problems in the workplace and recommends environmental adaptations. $50.00, 1/2" or 3/4" videotape format; includes brochures and discussion guide.

INDIVIDUALS WHO HAVE VISION LOSS AND HEARING LOSS

The number of individuals who are totally deaf and blind is relatively small. Individuals who are born deaf-blind require special education services and communication training. Those individuals who become deaf-blind during childhood, adolescence, or as adults often experience difficult emotional adjustment to sudden or unexpected severe loss.

With the increasing number of elders in our society, many more individuals are experiencing both hearing loss and vision loss, since both are age-related disabilities. It has been estimated that 30% of Americans 65 years or older have hearing impairments. (Hotchkiss: 1989). According to Bagley (1991), professionals in the aging field, health care professionals, and rehabilitation professionals need to make a concerted effort to work together to serve elders with dual sensory impairments. She suggests that service providers look beyond the narrow focus of the particular disability they are trained to work with; that self-help group referrals be specifically for groups of people with dual sensory impairments; and that elders have different types of goals than younger people who are involved in rehabilitation.

Service providers must take into account how these dual disabilities affect functioning. For example, people with vision loss and hearing loss may be unable to hear physicians' instructions for taking medications and may also be unable to read the instructions on bottles of medicine. Similarly, they may be unable to see oncoming traffic and unable to hear a horn or a companion's warning. A multidisciplinary rehabilitation plan will take into account both disabilities and train the individual in ways to compensate for these losses. Included in these plans must be primary care physicians, ophthalmologists, otologists, audiologists, and rehabilitation professionals.

State offices of vocational rehabilitation, private rehabilitation agencies, departments of otology and ophthalmology, as well as private practitioners offer services to individuals with hearing loss and vision loss. Some states have special agencies that serve people who are deaf or hearing impaired.

Many assistive devices are available for people with hearing loss. It is also possible to receive training in ways to make the most of remaining hearing and other senses. Professionals should be aware of how to facilitate communication with patients or clients who have experienced dual sensory losses. Rehabilitation professionals can demonstrate communication methods and assistive devices to other service providers. Special equipment, such as text telephones in offices and infrared listening devices in meeting halls, will help provide optimal services to individuals with hearing loss and vision loss.

144

References

Bagley, Martha
1991 "Older Adults with Vision and Hearing Losses" pp 71-91 in Susan L. Greenblatt, (ed.) Meeting the Needs of People with Vision Loss: A Multidisciplinary Perspective Lexington, MA: Resources for Rehabilitation

Hotchkiss, David
1989 The Hearing Impaired Elderly Population: Estimation, Projection, and Assessment, Monograph Series A, #1 Washington, D.C.: Gallaudet Research Institute

PROFESSIONAL ORGANIZATIONS

(In the listings below, telephone numbers have symbols V for voice and TT for text telephone where organizations have published this information.)

American Deafness and Rehabilitation Association (ADARA)
Box 55369
Little Rock, AR 722225
(501) 375-6643 (V/TT)

Organization for professionals and consumers that promotes services to deaf individuals. Publishes "Journal of American Deafness and Rehabilitation Association" and "ADARA Newsletter."

American Speech-Language-Hearing Association (ASHA)
10801 Rockville Pike
Rockville, MD 20852
(800) 638-8255   (301) 897-5700 (V/TT)

A professional organization of speech and language pathologists and audiologists. Provides information on hearing aids and communication problems and a FREE list of certified audiologists for each state.

Gallaudet Research Institute
Gallaudet University
800 Florida Avenue, NE
Washington, DC 20002
(202) 651-5400 (V/TT)

Conducts research on deafness and hearing impairment. Newsletter, "Research at Gallaudet," FREE.

National Institute on Deafness and Other Communication Disorders
National Institutes of Health
Building 31, Room 1B-62
9000 Rockville Pike
Bethesda, MD 20892
(301) 496-7243   (301) 492-0252 (TT)

Federal agency that funds basic research on hearing, balance, voice, language, and speech.

Rehabilitation Engineering Center of the Smith Kettlewell Eye Research Institute
2232 Webster Street
San Francisco, CA 94115
(415) 561-1619   FAX (415) 561-1610

A federally funded center that develops and tests new technology for individuals who are deaf-blind, visually impaired, or blind.

Rehabilitation Engineering Center on Technological Aids for Deaf and Hearing-Impaired Individuals
The Lexington Center
30th Avenue and 75th Street
Jackson Heights, NY 11370
(718) 899-8800   (718) 899-3030 (TT)   FAX (718) 899-9846

A federally funded center that studies technological aids for persons who are deaf or hearing impaired.

Research and Training Center on Deafness and Hearing Impairment
University of Arkansas
4601 West Markham Street
Little Rock, AR 72205
(501) 686-9691

A federally funded center that conducts surveys, develops training materials and curricula; and holds conferences.

Specialist to Older Adults
Helen Keller National Center for Deaf-Blind Youths and Adults (HKNC)
4455 LBJ Freeway, LB#3
Dallas, TX 75244-5998
(214) 490-9677 (V/TT)

Trains professionals who work with older adults who have hearing loss and vision loss. Sponsors national conferences.

Bagley, Martha
1989 <u>Identifying Vision and Hearing Problems Among Older Persons: Strategies and Resources</u> Helen Keller National Center for Deaf-Blind Youth and Adults, 111 Middle Neck Road, Sands Point, NY 11050

Functional Independence Training, Inc.
1990 <u>Resource Guide for Working with Deaf-Blind Persons</u> Functional Independence Training, Inc., 119 4th Street North, Suite 302D, Minneapolis, MN 55401

Luey, Helen Sloss, Dmitri Belser, and Laurel Glass
1989 <u>Beyond Refuge: Coping with Losses of Vision and Hearing in Late Life</u> Helen Keller National Center for Deaf-Blind Youth and Adults, 111 Middle Neck Road, Sands Point, NY 11050

Organizations

(In the listings below, telephone numbers have symbols V for voice and TT for text telephone where organizations have published this information.)

American Association of the Deaf-Blind (AADB)
814 Thayer Avenue, Room 300
Silver Spring, MD 20910
(301) 588-6545   (301) 523-1265 (TT)

A consumer organization, AADB advocates for coordinated services to individuals who are deaf-blind. Membership, $15.00, includes subscription to quarterly magazine, "The Deaf-Blind American," in LARGE PRINT and braille.

Canadian Deaf-Blind and Rubella Association
747 2nd Avenue East, Suite 4
Owen Sound, Ontario N4K 2G9 Canada
(519) 372-1333 (V/TT)   FAX (519) 372-1334

Develops training programs, conferences, and services for individuals who are deaf-blind, their families, and professionals. Eight chapters. Newsletter, "Intervention," published twice a year, in standard print and audiocassette. Membership, $15.00.

Helen Keller National Center for Deaf-Blind Youths and Adults (HKNC)
111 Middle Neck Road
Sands Point, NY 11050
(516) 944-8900 (V/TT)   FAX (516) 944-8751

Offers evaluation, rehabilitation, counseling, placement, and related services through eight regional offices. Sponsors national network of parents and state and local parent organizations. Newsletter, "HKNC TAC News," published three times a year in standard print, LARGE PRINT, and braille, FREE. HKNC's Specialist to Elderly Deaf-Blind Persons [4455 LBJ Freeway, LB#3, Suite 317, Dallas, TX 75244-5998, (214) 490-9677] provides services to professionals in the rehabilitation and aging fields.

National Information Center on Deafness
Gallaudet University
800 Florida Avenue, NE
Washington, DC 20002
(202) 651-5051   (202) 651-5052 (TT)   FAX (202) 651-5054

Provides information on education of deaf children, communication, hearing loss and aging, careers in deafness, and assistive devices. Many inexpensive or FREE publications.

RP Foundation Fighting Blindness
1401 Mt. Royal Avenue
Baltimore, MD 21217
(800) 683-5555   (410) 225-9400   (410) 225-9409 (TT)
FAX (410) 225-3936

Provides information about Usher Syndrome and makes referrals to Usher Syndrome Self-Help Network. Publishes "Information About Usher Syndrome" and a fact sheet, "Usher Syndrome Backgrounder." LARGE PRINT, FREE.

Self-Help for Hard of Hearing People (SHHH)
7800 Wisconsin Avenue
Bethesda, MD 20814
(301) 657-2248   (301) 657-2249 (TT)

Educates consumers and professionals about hearing loss. Makes referrals to local chapters, which hold self-help meetings. Holds an annual meeting. Membership, U.S., $15.00; Canada, $20.00; includes subscription to bimonthly magazine "SHHH" and discounts on other publications.

Usher Syndrome Project/Genetics
Boys Town National Research Hospital
555 North 30 Street
Omaha, NE 68131
(800) 835-1468 (V/TT)   In NE, (404) 498-6742

Conducts research to locate the gene(s) which cause Usher Syndrome. Families are needed to participate in the research.

Assistive Devices for Deaf-Blind Persons
Canadian National Institute for the Blind (CNIB)
1929 Bayview Avenue
Toronto, Ontario M4G 3E8 Canada
(416) 480-7580   FAX (416) 480-7677

Sells devices by mail. Request "Aids and Devices Catalog," standard print and braille. $20.00, Canadian funds.

Coping with Hearing Loss
by Susan V. Rezen and Carl Hausman
Dembner Books, NY

Discusses the causes of hearing loss, problems experienced by people with hearing loss, solutions for these problems, information about hearing aids, tips on lipreading, and a glossary. $15.95

Hearing and the Elderly
National Institute on Aging Information Center
PO Box 8057
Gaithersburg, MD 20898-8057
(301) 495-3455

Discusses common signs and types of hearing loss, treatment, and suggestions for communicating with people with hearing loss. LARGE PRINT, FREE.

I Work with a Guy Who's Deaf and Blind
Fanlight Productions
47 Halifax Street
Boston, MA 02130
(617) 524-0980   FAX (617) 524-8838

This videotape documents the accommodations a large company made for an employee who is deaf and blind. 11 minutes. Available in open and closed caption formats. Rental: $50.00 a day; $100.00 a week. Purchase: $125.00.

Living Skills: A Guide to Independence for Individuals with Deaf-blindness
Functional Independence Training, Inc. (FIND)
119 4th Street North, Suite 308
Minneapolis, MN 55401
(612) 333-9102 (V/TT)

Provides step-by-step instruction for activities of daily living such as food and nutrition, personal care, money management, and home care. Includes information on deaf-blindness, teaching, communication systems, and family life. Available in LARGE PRINT and braille. $35.00 plus shipping and handling.

Living with Hearing Loss
Resources for Rehabilitation
33 Bedford Street, Suite 19A
Lexington, MA 02173
(617) 862-6455   FAX (617) 861-7517

Designed for distribution by professionals, this LARGE PRINT (18 point bold type) publication describes a variety of organizations and publications that provide services to people with hearing loss. Minimum purchase, 25 copies. $2.00 per copy. Discounts available for purchases of 100 or more copies. See order form on last page of book.

Living with Low Vision
Resources for Rehabilitation
33 Bedford Street, Suite 19A
Lexington, MA 02173
(617) 862-6455   FAX (617) 861-7517

Designed for distribution by professionals, this LARGE PRINT (18 point bold type) publication describes a variety of organizations and publications that provide services to people with vision loss. Minimum purchase, 25 copies. $2.00 per copy. Discounts available for purchases of 100 or more copies. See order form on last page of book.

Resources for Elders with Disabilities
Resources for Rehabilitation
33 Bedford Street, Suite 19A
Lexington, MA 02173
(617) 862-6455   FAX (617) 861-7517

A LARGE PRINT resource directory describing services and products that elders with disabilities need to function independently. Includes chapters on vision loss, hearing loss, arthritis, diabetes, osteoporosis, Parkinson's disease, falls, and stroke. Updated biennially. $39.95 plus $5.00 shipping and handling.

Sound and Sight: Your Second Fifty Years
Lighthouse National Center on Vision and Aging (NCVA)
800 Second Avenue
New York, NY 10017
(800) 334-5497 (V/TT)   (212) 808-0077   FAX (212) 808-0110

A booklet that provides information on age-related hearing and vision loss and lists resources. $8.00. Also available, "Sound and Sight," a brochure which discusses loss of both vision and hearing in older adults. Available in English or Spanish; single copy, FREE.

Vision in Children - Normal and Abnormal
by Dr. Lea Hyvarinen
Canadian Deaf-Blind and Rubella Association
747 2nd Avenue East, Suite 4
Owen Sound, Ontario N4K 2G9 Canada
(519) 372-1333 (V/TT)   FAX (519) 372-1334

Compares visual development of children with normal vision and those with visual impairments; discusses the special needs of children with multiple disabilities; and recommends play and games for early motor development. Available in English and French. $7.00 (plus $2.50 for shipping outside Canada) Canadian funds.

The Department of Veterans Affairs (VA) has recognized that the increasing number of veterans with visual impairments require special care (Cohen et al.: 1987). The VA estimates that there are 60,000 to 100,000 blind veterans but, because legal blindness is not always identified or reported, the actual figure may be much larger (Evans: 1988).

The VA has identified legally blind veterans as a special interest group that requires a coordinated approach to services and has established the VIST (Visual Impairment Services Team) Program, available at many VA Medical Center throughout the country. All legally blind veterans eligible for VA services are eligible for VIST programs, whether their vision loss is service connected or not (Goodrich: 1991).

The ophthalmological assessment of a veteran's level of residual vision is crucial to the determination of compensation and pension benefits. However, legal blindness alone does not determine eligibility for AID and Attendance (A & A) status, a level of disability that may make a veteran eligible for a non-service connected VA pension. The VIST coordinator must assess other levels of disability to determine A & A status.

Veterans are eligible for a wide range of services. A booklet describing the benefits and rights of U.S. veterans, "Federal Benefits for Veterans and Dependents," is available for $2.75 from the Superintendent of Documents, U.S. Government Printing Office, Washington, DC 20402. Veterans with disabilities are eligible for counseling services and job assistance at Career Development Centers located in VA regional offices. These offices also offer a Vocational Rehabilitation and Counseling Service to help veterans with service-connected disabilities receive rehabilitation services and find employment.

The Department of Labor, local Veteran Employment Representatives, and Disabled Veteran Outreach Programs also provide services to disabled veterans. The U.S. Department of Education provides funding to institutions of higher education to conduct outreach programs to recruit veterans, including those with disabilities, and to provide counseling and tutoring. Contact the Assistant Secretary for Postsecondary Education, U.S. Department of Education, 400 Maryland Avenue, SW, Washington D.C. 20202

In October, 1990, the VA issued a legal interpretation that stated that mechanical or electronic equipment, which has been determined by appropriate authorities in the department to aid eligible veterans to "overcome the handicap of blindness," may be furnished by the department (Federal Register: October 10, 1990).

Five Blind Rehabilitation Centers offer comprehensive blindness rehabilitation programs for legally blind veterans with relatively good health and stamina. Three Blind Rehabilitation Clinics serve veterans who require slower-paced training programs due to physical or mental limitations. Veterans who are not legally blind (best corrected acuity is 20/50 to 20/200) are served by Vision Impairment Centers To Optimize Remaining Sight (VICTORS). VICTORS offers one-week, condensed, visual rehabilitation programs. (See listings below for locations.) Veterans who participate in any of these programs are provided with prosthetic and sensory aids free of charge upon completion of training.

References

Cohen, A.H., R. Soden, S.A. Martin, S. Liss, W.L.Hodson, and M. Meyer
1987 "A Comprehensive Eye/Vision Program" Journal of the American Optometric Association 58:386-389

Evans, Christopher J.
1988 "Managing and Training the Blind Veteran" VA Practitioner (May):41-51

Goodrich, Gregory L.
1991 "Low Vision Services in the VA: An Aging Trend" Journal of Vision Rehabilitation 5(3):11-17

Blind Rehabilitation Centers offer comprehensive blindness rehabilitation programs in a residential setting for legally blind veterans with relatively good health and stamina. Enrollment at the centers is free and in some cases, the VA may pay for the veterans' travel costs.

Participants receive training in orientation and mobility and skills of daily living; counseling; and a low vision evaluation. Each Blind Rehabilitation Center has an independent living program for those veterans who will be living alone after rehabilitation. The length of the training program depends upon the individual's needs, but usually ranges from eight to sixteen weeks.

There are five blindness rehabilitation centers in the U.S. Regional consultants from each center travel to VA Medical Centers within the region. Contact the VIS Team coordinator at the nearest VA Medical Center to obtain more specific information about the program.

Central Blind Rehabilitation Center
VA Hospital (124)
Hines, IL 60141
(708) 216-2272   FAX (708) 381-2721

Eastern Blind Rehabilitation Center
VA Medical Center
950 Campbell Avenue
West Haven, CT 06516
(203) 932-5711   FAX (203) 428-3878

San Juan Blind Rehabilitation Center
VA Medical Center (124)
1 Veterans Plaza
San Juan, PR 00927-5800
(809) 758-7575, extension 4023   FAX (809) 766-6027

Southeastern Blind Rehabilitation Center
VA Medical Center (124)
700 South 19th Street
Birmingham, AL 35233
(205) 933-8101   FAX (205) 933-4484

Western Blind Rehabilitation Center
VA Medical Center (124)
3801 Miranda Boulevard
Palo Alto, CA 94304
(415) 493-5000   FAX (415) 463-4700

BLIND REHABILITATION CLINICS

Blind Rehabilitation Clinics serve veterans who require slower-paced training programs due to additional physical conditions or mental limitations. The following VA Medical Center house Blind Rehabilitation Clinics.

American Lake Blind Rehabilitation Clinic
VA Medical Center (124)
American Lake
Tacoma, WA 98493
(206) 582-8440, extension 6200   FAX (206) 396-6239

Eastern Blind Rehabilitation Clinic
VA Medical Center (124)
950 Campbell Avenue
West Haven, CT 06516
(203) 932-5711   FAX (203) 428-3878

Waco Blind Rehabilitation Clinic
VA Medical Center (124)
4800 Memorial Drive
Waco, TX 76711
(817) 752-6581   FAX (817) 734-6332

VICTORS

Veterans who are not legally blind (best corrected acuity is 20/40 or less) are served by Vision Impairment Centers To Optimize Remaining Sight (VICTORS). VICTORS offers three to five day visual rehabilitation programs which provide low vision evaluations, individual and family counseling, rehabilitation training, and low vision devices.

VICTORS Programs are available at these locations:

Northport VA Medical Center
Building 2 (123)
Northport, NY 11768
(516) 261-4400, extension 2068

VA Medical Center
Eye/VICTORS Clinic (112G)
4801 East Linwood Boulevard
Kansas City, MO 64128
(816) 861-4700, extension 661

VA West Side Medical Center
820 South Damen Avenue
Chicago, IL 60612
(312) 666-6500, extension 3505
In IL and outside Chicago, (800) 537-8297

Organizations

(In the listings below, telephone numbers have symbols V for voice and TT for text telephone where organizations have published this information.)

Blinded Veterans Association (BVA)
477 H Street, NW
Washington, DC 20001-2694
(800) 669-7079   (202) 371-8880

The BVA's field service and outreach employment programs help veterans find rehabilitation services, training, and employment. Offers scholarships to spouses and dependent children of blinded veterans. Membership, $8.00, includes the "BVA Bulletin" in LARGE PRINT and on disc.

Canadian National Institute for the Blind
1931 Bayview Avenue
Toronto, Ontario M4G 4C8 Canada
(416) 480-7580   FAX (416) 480-7677

Provides services to war-blinded and blind veterans.

Disabled American Veterans (DAV)
807 Maine Avenue, SW
Washington, DC 20024
(202) 554-3501

DAV National Service Officers advocate for veterans and their families. Provides transportation to VA Medical Centers and emergency relief for veterans with financial crises. Provides scholarships for children of eligible disabled veterans. National DAV Blind Chapter. Membership, $15.00, includes "DAV Magazine," available in standard print and audiocassette; nonmember subscription, $4.00.

State Offices of Veterans Affairs

States also provide veterans' services. In some states, special benefits are available to veterans with service-connected blindness. The state government information operator can direct callers to state offices of veterans affairs.

Coordinated Services for Blinded Veterans
Veterans Health Administration
Blind Rehabilitation Service
810 Vermont Avenue, NW
Washington, DC 20420

Describes the services provided at blind rehabilitation centers and clinics. Available in LARGE PRINT. FREE

Federal Benefits for Veterans and Dependents
Consumer Information Center 2B
PO Box 100
Pueblo, CO 81002.

Describes the benefits available under federal laws. $2.75

Talking American Legion Magazine
American Legion
PO Box 1055
Indianapolis, IN 46206

Published monthly on four-track audiocassette. FREE

A Summary of Department of Veterans Affairs Benefits

Available from any VA regional office. FREE

Chapter 6

EMPLOYMENT FOR PEOPLE WITH VISION LOSS

For many individuals with irreversible vision loss, the fear of losing their jobs is para-mount. It is important that these individuals understand, that in many cases, they can continue in their chosen careers, often with the help of adaptive equipment. For those individuals with vision loss who are in careers which require excellent vision, such as airplane pilots or surgeons, retraining or additional education may open up new fields of endeavor.

Individuals who are experiencing vision loss but who are not legally blind (a requirement for vocational rehabilitation in many states) should not wait for their eye disease or condition to progress to legal blindness before seeking vocational help. Many types of accommodations can be made to help them retain their jobs, including adaptive aids, changes in responsibilities and schedules, and trade-offs with other employees. Professionals who make referrals for vocational rehabilitation as well as professionals who actually provide vocational rehabilitation services should not assume that older individuals do not want to continue working.

An assessment of the individual's current work environment and tasks by a qualified vocational rehabilitation counselor will help to determine if the individual will be able to stay in his or her current position with modifications or if retraining for a different position is required. Those individuals who are not eligible for state services should be referred to a private rehabilitation counselor. Some individuals have progressive diseases that may cause their vision to decrease as time passes. Examples of these diseases are retinitis pigmentosa and macular degeneration. These individuals may need to have their work environment modified as their vision deteriorates.

Many employers are able to help people with vision loss and other disabilities retain their positions or find another suitable position in the same organization through the efforts of the affirmative action office. On July 26, 1990, the *Americans with Disabilities Act* (ADA) was passed. Considered the most important piece of civil rights legislation in recent years, the ADA (P.L 101-336) increases the steps employers must take to accommodate employees with disabilities. According to the law, an individual with a disability is a person who has a physical or mental impairment that substantially limits one or more major activities; someone who has had such an impairment; or someone who is regarded as having such an impairment. Disabilities include chronic conditions such as cancer, epilepsy, and AIDS and disfigurements. Although the definition of disability is very broad, it is based upon previous legislation (such as the Rehabilitation Act) and a large body of case law.

The ADA prohibits discrimination against individuals with disabilities who are otherwise qualified to carry out the essential functions of a position, with or without reasonable

Rehabilitation Resource Manual: VISION Lexington, MA: Resources for Rehabilitation, copyright 1993

accommodations. The employer determines what is considered to be the essential functions of the position by writing a job description prior to advertising the position. "Reasonable accommodations" include making existing facilities accessible or job restructuring, which means reassignment to a different position; modification or provision of equipment; training; or provision of interpreters and readers.

Discrimination is defined as limiting the opportunities of a job applicant or employee; engaging in an arrangement with a referral agency, union, or other organization that discriminates against individuals with disabilities; not making reasonable accommodations for an applicant or employee; using tests or other screening criteria that eliminate individuals with disabilities, unless the criteria are job related; failing to administer tests to individuals with disabilities in the most effective manner to accommodate the disability, unless the disability would prevent the person from carrying out the essential functions of the job. Inquiries about a disability and pre-employment medical examinations are prohibited prior to the conditional offer of employment; questions related to the ability to carry out job functions are allowed. Medical examinations may be conducted following a conditional offer of employment only if all employees, including those without disabilities, are required to undergo such examinations. Information collected about disabilities must be kept confidential except to inform supervisors about necessary work restrictions and accommodations regarding safety and first aid.

Employers are protected from "undue hardship" in complying with the ADA. The financial situation of the employer and the size and type of business are considered when determining whether an accommodation would constitute "undue hardship." Employers with 25 or more employees must comply with the law by July 26, 1992; employers with 15 to 24 must comply by July 26, 1994.

Remedies available to employees or job candidates who believe that their employment rights under the ADA have been violated are those specified under Title VII of the Civil Rights Act of 1964. Administrative enforcement by the Equal Employment Opportunity Commission is the first level of enforcement. After administrative appeals have been exhausted, the right to sue in the federal courts is permitted. Employers violating the law are subject to fines, injunctions ordering compliance, and both back pay and future pay for the individuals who have proved discrimination. The enforcement is coordinated with the enforcement of the Rehabilitation Act of 1973 in order to prevent duplication of effort.

Section 503 of the *Rehabilitation Act* requires any contractor that receives more than $2,500 in contracts from the federal government to take affirmative action to employ individuals with disabilities. The Office of Federal Contract Compliance Programs within the Department of Labor is responsible for enforcing this provision (see "ORGANIZATIONS" section below). Section 504 requires that federal agencies develop an affirmative action plan for hiring, placing, and promoting individuals with disabilities and for making their facilities accessible. The Civil Rights Division of the Department of Justice is responsible for enforcing this section.

VOCATIONAL REHABILITATION

In the U.S., a vocational rehabilitation agency (often called "voc rehab" or "VR") in each state is responsible for training or retraining individuals with disabilities to become employable, independent, and integrated into the community. In some states, there are two vocational rehabilitation agencies; one that serves individuals who are visually impaired or blind and another that serves individuals with other types of disabilities. In other states, one agency serves people with all types of disabilities, including vision impairment and blindness. Vocational rehabilitation services are offered at locations throughout the state. Consult the state listing in the telephone book for a local vocational rehabilitation office or contact the main office listed in Appendix A: State Agencies for Individuals Who Are Visually Impaired or Blind.

When individuals have a visual impairment that entitles them to vocational rehabilitation services, federal law requires that they and a vocational rehabilitation counselor jointly develop an Individualized Written Rehabilitation Plan (IWRP) that specifies employment goals and the services to be provided by the vocational rehabilitation agency. Both the individual and the counselor must sign the IWRP, which may be amended or modified with reasonable justification and agreement by both parties. The vocational rehabilitation agency's Client Assistance Program (CAP) will provide assistance in solving any problems encountered in obtaining vocational rehabilitation services.

Vocational rehabilitation services are provided until the individual is successfully rehabilitated or until a determination is made that a goal cannot be reached. A case may not be closed until the individual has been suitably and satisfactorily employed for at least 60 days.

Individuals who are visually impaired or blind fare relatively well in the federally funded vocational rehabilitation services. According to a recent report (General Accounting Office: 1991), clients who were visually impaired received the second highest mean number of services and the services they received cost more than services provided to clients with any other type of disability.

OTHER PROGRAMS

Projects with Industry (PWI's) are cooperative ventures between employers and private organizations which serve individuals with disabilities. PWI's facilitate employment through referral of qualified applicants for suitable positions, consultation on accessibility issues, and employer training programs. Further information is available from the regional office of the Rehabilitation Services Administration, U.S. Department of Education.

The Social Security Administration's PASS Program, or Plan to Achieve Self Support, provides incentives for people with disabilities to return to work. It allows recipients of

Supplemental Social Security Income to set aside income and resources for a specific time period while working to achieve an employment oriented goal. These goals may include education, starting a business, or obtaining adaptive equipment. The Social Security Administration provides information on this program through its toll-free number [(800) 772-1213 or (800) 325-0778 for TT users].

Federal Job Information Centers, listed under "U.S. Government" in metropolitan area telephone directories, provide information about jobs in federal service and help individuals apply for these positions. Some federal job screening tests are available in LARGE PRINT, braille, or recorded formats; the Job Information Center must provide a reader if special formats are unavailable. Assistance to individuals with disabilities is also available through selective placement coordinators at all federal agencies.

The Small Business Administration (SBA) offers Federal assistance and low cost loans to individuals with disabilities who are interested in starting their own businesses. The SBA toll-free information line will provide individuals with information about this program [(800) 368-5855].

Many states promote employment through a Governor's Committee on Employment of People with Disabilities, which sponsors training programs, job fairs, publications, and other awareness activities.

The Canadian National Institute for the Blind (See "Appendix B: Division Offices of the Canadian National Institute for the Blind") and private agencies that serve individuals who are visually impaired or blind also offer career development and employment services.

ENVIRONMENTAL ADAPTATIONS

The work environment may be made accessible for employees who are visually impaired or blind, often without great effort or expense. Simple modifications will result in less anxiety for people with vision loss, and co-workers will be less concerned about them falling or bumping into objects. Two obvious examples are providing good lighting and eliminating all possible sources of glare.

Elevators should have braille or raised numerals to indicate floors; taped announcements of the floor number are also helpful. Some people with vision loss also have other disabilities and may use walkers, canes, scooters, or wheelchairs for mobility. Corridors and aisles should be wide enough to accommodate these mobility aids and should be cleared of clutter and projecting objects.

When designing or remodeling an office, the needs of employees with vision loss should be a major concern. Contrasting colors should be used for carpeting, furniture, and walls. Placing yellow tape or painting stripes on the edge of steps helps people with visual impairment navigate. A metal edge on a carpeted step or a change in the texture of the flooring will provide tactile cues for individuals who are blind. Doors should be kept either closed or completely open. Chairs should be replaced under tables or desks. Partially-open doors and chairs left in the middle of a room are dangerous.

Personnel forms and office procedure manuals should be made available in LARGE PRINT, audiocassette, or braille. Signs should have large letters and good contrast. Telephones should be adapted with LARGE PRINT numerals for easy use by individuals who are visually impaired. Employees who are totally blind may find that raised dots on the 4-5-6 row of a telephone will guide them when dialing. Similarly, raised dots on the "f" and "j" keys of a keyboard will help when typing.

Individuals who are totally blind or who have light perception only will require different types of adaptations than individuals who retain useful vision. These individuals will often use braille to read and write documents, although they use regular computer keyboards as well. Although sighted co-workers are probably unable to read and write braille, computers that are designed to be used with braille also transcribe the data into written output.

Additional suggestions made throughout this book for environmental adaptations to the home and to professional service providers' offices may be applicable to the workplace as well.

References

General Accounting Office
1991 Vocational Rehabilitation Program: Client Characteristics, Services Received, and Employment Outcomes Washington, D.C.: General Accounting Office

Roy Jordan: Work Modifications for Progressive Vision Loss

Roy Jordan was diagnosed with retinitis pigmentosa several years ago. Until recently, his only vision problem had been night blindness. Since he commutes by train to his job in the city, traveling home during the winter months had become difficult. Several of his neighbors take the same train and therefore, he usually has a companion who helps him by offering sighted guide on the walk home from the train station.

Recently, Mr. Jordan has noticed that his vision seems worse during daylight hours. Sometimes he does not recognize fellow workers in the cafeteria or at meetings; he occasionally bumps into things at home and in the office; and the other day, he was almost hit by a bicyclist as he started to cross the street near the office. He is also finding that his reading speed is slower; he has to continually move his head back and forth because he can only see a few words at a time. The computer screen he uses is very bright and the glare interferes with his work. These problems are causing him to have trouble meeting deadlines, and he is worried about losing his job.

Mr. Jordan scheduled an appointment with his ophthalmologist, Dr. Linda Goodhart, and discussed these problems. Dr. Goodhart examined Mr. Jordan, performed several tests, and confirmed that Mr. Jordan's visual fields had indeed decreased by several degrees. Although Mr. Jordan was not yet legally blind and therefore not eligible for services from the state agency that serves individuals who are visually impaired or blind, Dr. Goodhart discussed with Mr. Jordan the need to prepare for progressive vision loss. She told Mr. Jordan about the many services and types of equipment, including computers with speech output, that could enable him to continue working once his vision is no longer adequate to use standard computer equipment. She encouraged Mr. Jordan to return to her office whenever he notices a change in his vision; these visits would enable Dr. Goodhart to refer Mr. Jordan to the state agency as soon as he becomes eligible. In the meantime, Dr. Goodhart suggested that Mr. Jordan contact the local chapter of the RP Foundation Fighting Blindness, which sponsors support groups for people with RP, at all stages of the disease. She gave Mr. Jordan the name and phone number of the local coordinator for the support group.

Continued on next page

At the first meeting he attended of the RP support group, Mr. Jordan introduced himself and explained the problems that he was encountering. One group member suggested that life becomes much easier when a person with RP explains to friends and colleagues at work the types of vision problems that are occurring and why it is difficult to recognize familiar faces. Another member of the group, who had had similar problems several months earlier, suggested a program in which a consultant visits the job site, assesses the client's visual needs and makes recommendations for adaptations. Mr. Jordan accepted this information, although he was nervous about drawing attention to his problems at work. After several days of pondering the situation, Mr. Jordan decided that if he did not make some changes, he would lose his job, so he asked his supervisor to approve the consultant's visit. His supervisor, who had noticed the change in Mr. Jordan's work, was supportive, and an appointment was made for the consultant to visit the office.

The consultant, Freda Sharp, recommended that Mr. Jordan take lessons in orientation and mobility, in order to travel on his own safely and reduce the likelihood of accidents indoors as well. She also advised that fellow employees take care in keeping aisles clear of clutter and protruding objects. Mr. Jordan agreed to enlist the help of an orientation and mobility instructor. Ms Sharp also suggested that Mr. Jordan use a different combination of colors on his computer monitor. After experimenting, he found that white print on black reduced the glare sufficiently. A contrast enhancement filter adhered to the monitor with velcro strips increased his comfort. Ms Sharp also suggested that he use a line marker on the text to help him keep his place. Some of the features of regular word processing programs, such as scrolling, windowing, and a larger cursor, also proved helpful. Ms Sharp suggested that a speech program might help reduce stress by confirming what Mr. Jordan has just typed and allowing him to hear the finished document rather than struggling to read it phrase by phrase. Mr. Jordan recalled Dr. Goodhart's reference to computers with speech output, but Dr. Goodhart had not thought that Mr. Jordan needed this equipment yet. Therefore, Mr. Jordan decided to wait to purchase an additional piece of computer equipment, since the state agency may pay for this equipment or lend it to him at no cost when he becomes eligible for state services.

Following the consultation, Ms Sharp wrote up a summary of her suggestions and sent them to both Mr. Jordan and his supervisor. She reminded both of them that if Mr. Jordan's vision continues to decrease, he should be reassessed for additional modifications.

(In the listings below, telephone numbers have symbols V for voice and TT for text telephone where organizations have published this information.)

American Bar Association (ABA)
1800 M Street, NW
Washington, DC 20036-5886
(202) 331-2240   FAX (202) 331-2220

Operates the ABA Research Services and Disability Law Network, which enables professionals to search a variety of databases with laws, legal cases, and recent developments in the field of disability. Also maintains an Americans with Disabilities Act database of articles, Congressional debates, and cases. Publishes the "Mental and Physical Disability Law Reporter" six times per year, which covers legal cases related to disability and entitlement and reviews federal and state legislation. Individual subscription, $183.00; agency subscription, $238.00.

Mainstream, Inc.
3 Bethesda Metro Center, Suite 830
Bethesda, MD 20814
(301) 654-2400 (V/TT)

Provides training and technical assistance, publishes reference guides, and sponsors annual conference to advocate for employment of people with disabilities.

National Association of Rehabilitation Professionals in the Private Sector (NARPPS)
PO Box 697
Brookline, MA 02146
(617) 566-4432

A membership organization of rehabilitation professionals who are self-employed or work for private organizations. Publishes a biennial directory of members.

National Federation of the Blind (NFB)
1800 Johnson Street
Baltimore, MD 21230
(410) 659-9314   FAX (410) 685-5653

Operates the Information Access Project for Blind Individuals, funded by the U.S. Department of Justice, to educate local and state governments as well as private employers about the Americans with Disabilities Act as it applies to individuals who are blind. Provides technical assistance in making text available in nonvisual media. Also performs brailling services.

National Rehabilitation Association (NRA)
1910 Association Drive, Suite 205
Reston, VA 22091
(703) 715-9090   (703) 715-9209 (TT)   FAX (703) 715-1058

Membership organization for professionals who work in the field of vocational rehabilitation. Includes a division called the National Association of Service Providers in Private Rehabilitation. Holds annual training conference. Membership benefits include "Journal of Rehabilitation" and "NRA Newsletter."

PROFESSIONAL PUBLICATIONS

A Guide for Managers and Supervisors on the Employment of People with Disabilities in the Federal Government Equal Employment Opportunity Commission, 1801 L Street, NW, 10th floor, Washington, DC 20507

Job Accommodation Handbook RPM Press, PO Box 31483, Tucson, AZ 85751-1483

Journal of Applied Rehabilitation Counseling, National Rehabilitation Counseling Association, 1910 Association Drive, Suite 205, Reston, VA 22091

Journal of Rehabilitation, National Rehabilitation Association, 1910 Association Drive, Suite 205, Reston, VA 22091

Journal of Vocational Rehabilitation, Andover Medical Publishers, 80 Montvale Avenue, Stoneham, MA 02180

Mental and Physical Disability Law Reporter American Bar Association Commission on the Mentally Disabled, 1800 M Street, NW, Suite 200, Washington, DC 20036

Mueller, James
1990 The Workplace Workbook Washington, DC: RESNA Press, Department 4813, Washington, DC 20061-4813

Rehabilitation Psychology, Springer Publishing, 536 Broadway, New York, NY 10012

Rubin, Stanford E., and Richard T. Roessler
1987 Foundations of Vocational Rehabilitation Process Austin, TX: Pro-Ed

Work, Andover Medical Publishers, 80 Montvale Avenue, Stoneham, MA 02180

Organizations

(In the listings below, telephone numbers have symbols V for voice and TT for text telephone where organizations have published this information.)

Architectural and Transportation Barriers Compliance Board (ATBCB)
1331 F Street, NW, Suite 1000
Washington, DC 20004-1111
(800) 872-2253 (V/TT)   (202) 272-5434   (202) 272-5449 (TT)
FAX (202) 272-5447

A federal agency charged with developing standards for accessibility in federal facilities, public accommodations, and transportation facilities as required by the Americans with Disabilities Act and other federal laws. Provides technical assistance, sponsors research, and distributes publications. Publishes a quarterly newsletter, "Access America." Publications available in standard print, LARGE PRINT, audiocassette, computer disk, and braille. FREE

Breaking New Ground Resource Center
Purdue University
1146 Agricultural Engineering Building
West Lafayette, IN 47907-1146
(317) 494-5088 (V/TT)   FAX (317) 496-1115

Provides assistance to farmers with disabilities in areas such as career decisions, assistive technology, and resources. Publishes "Breaking New Ground" newsletter, FREE. Produces "Plowshares Technical Reports," with titles such as "Farming with a Visual Impairment," "Alternative Farm Enterprises for Farmers with Disabilities," and "Rural Public Libraries: A Resource for the Disabled." FREE

Computer/Electronic Accommodations Program (CAP)
Department of Defense
Defense Medical Systems Support Center
5109 Leesburg Pike, Suite 502
Falls Church, VA 22041-3201
(703) 756-8811 (V/TT)

Assists Department of Defense in meeting accessibility requirements through information on technology and disability management issues. Publishes "News Bulletin," in standard print, disk, and braille. FREE

Department of Justice
Civil Rights Division
PO Box 66118
Washington, DC 20035-6118
(202) 514-0301 (V)   (202) 514-0381 (TT)   (202) 514-0383 (TT)

Responsible for enforcing the Americans with Disabilities Act and sections 503 and 504 of the Rehabilitation Act. Copies of its regulations are available in standard print, LARGE PRINT, braille, computer disk, audiocassette, and on an electronic bulletin board, (202) 514-6193.

Department of Labor
Office of Federal Contract Compliance Programs (OFCCP)
Employment Standards Administration
200 Constitution Avenue, NW, Room C-3325
Washington, DC 20210
(202) 523-9476   FAX (202) 523-0195

Reviews contractors' affirmative action plans, provides technical assistance to contractors, investigates complaints and resolves issues between contractors and employees. Ten regional offices throughout the country serve as liaisons with the national office and with district offices under their jurisdiction.

Disability Rights Education and Defense Fund (DREDF)
2212 Sixth Street
Berkeley, CA 94710
(415) 644-2555   (415) 644-2626 (TT)

Provides technical assistance, information, and referrals on laws and rights; provides legal representation in both individual and class action cases related to employment, education, transportation, and accessibility; trains law students, parents, and legislators.

Equal Employment Opportunity Commission (EEOC)
1801 L Street, NW, 10th floor
Washington, DC 20507
Recorded messages in English and Spanish; order publications and forms to file complaints; and option to speak with an EEOC employee:
(800) 669-3362 for calls from touch tone phones
(800) 669-4000 for calls from rotary dial phones
(800) 800-3302 (TT)

Responsible for developing and enforcing regulations for the employment section of the ADA. Copies of its regulations are available in standard print, LARGE PRINT, audiocassette, computer disk, and braille.

4-Sights Network
Greater Detroit Society for the Blind
16625 Grand River Avenue
Detroit, MI 48227
(313) 272-3900

A computer bulletin board with information on products, rehabilitation, and ADA resources. No user fee other than telephone charges. Phone (313) 272-7111 and log in as "newuser." The "Occupational Information Library for the Blind" provides a vocational information reference guide for employers and potential employees. Lists nearly 500 types of jobs held by people with vision loss, the education and training required, adaptive aids, and employment future.

Hadley School for the Blind
700 Elm Street
Winnetka, IL 60093
(800) 323-4238   In IL, (708) 446-8111

Offers correspondence courses on careers and employment for individuals who are legally blind, have a prognosis of legal blindness, or are hearing impaired with a prognosis of vision loss. Requires ability to read and understand high school level courses. FREE. Course catalogue available in LARGE PRINT, audiocassette, and braille. FREE

Internal Revenue Service (IRS)
(800) 829-3676   (800) 829-4059 (TT)
(202) 566-3292 information for business requirements under the ADA

To receive Publication 501, "Exemptions, Standard Deduction, and Filing Information," Publication 907, "Tax Information for Persons with Handicaps or Disabilities," and Publication 524, "Credit for the Elderly or the Disabled," call the number listed above.

Job Accommodation Network (JAN)
West Virginia University
809 Allen Hall, PO Box 6122
Morgantown, WV 26506-6122
(800) 526-7234   In WV, (800) 526-4698   In Canada, (800) 526-2262

Maintains database of products that facilitate accommodation in the workplace. Provides information to employers about practical accommodations which enable them to employ individuals with disabilities.

Job Opportunities for the Blind (JOB)
National Federation of the Blind (NFB)
1800 Johnson Street
Baltimore, MD 21230
(800) 638-7518   In MD, (410) 659-9314   FAX (410) 685-5653

A nationwide employment service available to any person who is legally blind and to employers seeking job candidates. Provides literature on job seeking strategies, FREE.

National Industries for the Blind (NIB)
524 Hamburg Turnpike, CN969
Wayne, NJ 07474-0969
(201) 595-9200

Conducts a six month internship program for individuals who are legally blind and are seeking professional employment. Requires that candidates have a bachelor's degree in a field related to business or communications and a grade point average of 3.0. Provides stipend, housing, and relocation expenses plus job accommodations. Interns work in one of NIB's offices or industrial facilities.

National Resume Database for Students with Disabilities
Association on Higher Education and Disability (AHEAD)
PO Box 21192
Columbus, OH 43221-0192
(614) 488-4972 (V/TT)   FAX (614) 488-1174

A database that enables students with disabilities to disseminate their resumes to potential employers. The employer receives information about the students' qualifications, not their disabilities. It is up to the student and employer to discuss accommodations. Students may obtain a database form by sending a self-addressed, stamped envelope to AHEAD. Forms may also be available in disabled student service offices on campus. No charge for students. Employers interested in purchasing or searching the database should contact Resume Link, PO Box 218, Hilliard, OH 43026 (614) 771-7087

President's Committee on Employment of People with Disabilities (PCEPD)
1331 F Street, NW
Washington, DC 20004
(202) 376-6200   (202) 376-6205 (TT)   FAX (202) 376-6219

Advocates on behalf of people with disabilities, holds an annual conference, and sponsors studies. All publications, including "Worklife," a quarterly magazine, and "Newsbrief," a newsletter, are available in standard print, LARGE PRINT, audiocassette, and braille. FREE

Rehabilitation Services Administration (RSA)
Department of Education
400 Maryland Avenue, SW
Washington, DC 20202
(202) 205-5482   FAX (202) 205-9874

Responsible for administering the Rehabilitation Act. Provides funding for state vocational rehabilitation programs and the Projects with Industry Program.

Small Business Administration
409 Third Street, SW
Washington, DC 20416
(800) 827-5722

Direct loan funds up to $150,000 available to applicants, including individuals with disabilities and disabled and Vietnam-era veterans. Must be unable to secure SBA-guaranteed loan. List of SBA publications and videotapes on small business operations are available from the Small Business Directory, PO Box 1000, Fort Worth, TX 76119.

Social Security Administration
6401 Security Boulevard
Baltimore, MD 21235
(800) 772-1213   (800) 325-0778 (TT)

To apply for Social Security benefits based on disability or Medicare, call the number above to set up an appointment with a Social Security representative, or visit the Social Security office nearest you. The Office of Disability within the Social Security Administration publishes "Social Security Regulations: Rules for Determining Disability and Blindness," FREE.

American Rehabilitation
Superintendent of Documents
U.S. Government Printing Office
Washington, DC 20402

Published by the Rehabilitation Services Administration, this magazine provides information on rehabilitation programs, services, and publications. Published quarterly, U.S., $5.00; foreign, $6.25.

Blind Workers
Lions Clubs International, Public Relations Division
300 22nd Street
Oak Brook, IL 60521
(708) 571-5466

Videotape describes new technology and training that enable people who are visually impaired or blind to continue working. 23 minutes. Videotape (VHS or Beta) $25.00; 16mm film $100.00

Career Perspectives: Interviews with Blind and Visually Impaired Professionals
American Foundation for the Blind (AFB)
15 West 16th Street
New York, NY 10011
(800) 232-5463   (212) 620-2000   FAX (212) 620-2105

Twenty professionals discuss their experiences preparing for and obtaining employment. LARGE PRINT, audiocassette, and braille. $11.95 plus $3.00 shipping and handling.

Careers & the Disabled
Equal Opportunity Publications
44 Broadway
Greenlawn, NY 11740
(516) 261-8899

Offers career guidance articles and role-model profiles; lists companies seeking qualified job candidates. Published twice a year, $10.00.

The Careers Catalogue
Department of Rehabilitation
Canadian National Institute for the Blind (CNIB)
1931 Bayview Avenue
Toronto, Ontario M4G 4C8 Canada
(416) 480-7626   FAX (416) 480-7677

Describes more than 175 jobs in the public and private sectors that are carried out by individuals who are visually impaired or blind. Describes job tasks and job accommodations used. Available in standard print and audiocassette. $19.95, Canadian funds.

Careers: Job Searching and Success
National Library for the Blind and Physically Handicapped (NLS)
1291 Taylor Street, NW
Washington, DC 20542
(800) 424-8567 or 8572 (Reference Section)
(800) 424-9100 (to receive application)
(202) 707-5100   FAX (202) 707-0712

A bibliography of materials on disc, audiocassette, and braille that describe career options and job searching skills. Materials listed are available through the NLS regional libraries. FREE

Employment of Persons with Physical Impairments or Mental Retardation in the Federal Service
Office of Personnel Management
Washington, DC 20415-0001

Describes federal employment opportunities for individuals with disabilities through competitive appointment or special appointing authorities and special accommodations for examination procedures and on the job. FREE

Meeting the Needs of Employees with Disabilities
Resources for Rehabilitation
33 Bedford Street, Suite 19A
Lexington, MA 02173
(617) 862-6455   FAX (617) 861-7517

Provides information to help people with disabilities retain or obtain employment. Chapters on vision, mobility, and hearing and speech impairments include information on organizations, products, and services. $42.95 plus $5.00 shipping and handling. See order form on last page of this book.

Opening Doors: Blind and Visually Impaired People and Work
Department of Rehabilitation
Canadian National Institute for the Blind (CNIB)
1931 Bayview Avenue
Toronto, Ontario M4G 4C8 Canada
(416) 480-7626   FAX (416) 480-7677

Surveys Canadian and international literature on the subject of employment for persons with vision loss. Available in standard print and audiocassette. $21.95, Canadian funds.

Red Book on Work Incentives
A Summary Guide to Social Security and Supplemental Security Income Work Incentives for People with Disabilities
Social Security Administration

Overview of work incentives for individuals who receive SSDI or SSI. Includes impairment-related work expenses, trial work period, continuation of Medicare coverage, earned income exclusion, and other work incentives. LARGE PRINT. Request SSA Publication 64-030 through Social Security Administration Regional Office listed in telephone directory under U.S. government. FREE

Take Charge: a Strategic Guide for Blind Job Seekers
National Braille Press (NBP)
88 St. Stephen Street
Boston, MA 02115
(617) 266-6160   FAX (617) 437-0456

This book includes examples of the strategies used by successfully employed individuals. Available in standard print, four-track audiocassette, IBM disk (5 1/4" and 3 1/2"), VersaBraille II+ disk (3 1/2") and braille. $19.95 (add $4.00 shipping for print edition).

Work Sight
Braille Institute of America, Inc.
741 North Vermont Avenue
Los Angeles, CA 90029-9988
(800) 272-4553

Individuals who are visually impaired describe their transition to the workplace in this video. Emotional and psychological adjustments as well as a team approach to solving problems are discussed. $25.00

<u>Work Sight</u>
Lighthouse National Center for Vision and Aging (NCVA)
800 Second Avenue
New York, NY 10017
(800) 334-5497 (V/TT)   (212) 808-0077   FAX (212) 808-0110

This videotape discusses age-related vision problems in the workplace and recommends environmental adaptations. $50.00, 1/2" or 3/4" video format; includes brochures and discussion guide.

Many people with low vision continue to work by using "high-tech" electronic aids. These aids include closed circuit television systems (CCTV's) and computers with LARGE PRINT, speech, or braille output.

Computer access centers have been established at many public libraries and universities, where individuals may see the equipment and have "hands-on" experience before purchasing their own equipment. Some libraries will lend portable equipment to patrons.

The Technology Related Assistance for Individuals with Disabilities Act (P.L. 100-407) was passed in 1988 and provides grants to states to develop model systems for the delivery of assistive technology; conduct needs assessments; support training activities for professionals and for individuals with disabilities; and to conduct public awareness campaigns.

PROFESSIONAL ORGANIZATIONS

(In the listings below, telephone numbers have symbols V for voice and TT for text telephone where organizations have published this information.)

Connecticut Rehabilitation Engineering Center for Technology Resources
78 Eastern Boulevard
Glastonbury, CT 06033
(203) 657-9954   (203) 657-8418 (TT)   FAX (203) 657-9032

A federally funded research center that develops, demonstrates, and disseminates technology for people with disabilities. Evaluates service delivery models, conducts continuing education programs, and develops databases.

Electronic Industries Foundation (EIF)
919 18th Street, Suite 900
Washington, DC 20006
(202) 955-5810   (202) 955-5836 (TT)   FAX (202) 955-5837

EIF's Rehabilitation Engineering Center for Rehabilitation Technology Transfer encourages the participation of industry in the development and distribution of assistive technology.

Office of Opportunities in Science
American Association for the Advancement of Science (AAAS)
1333 H Street, NW
Washington, DC 20005
(202) 326-6667 (V/TT)

A network of support for scientists with disabilities. Publishes "Resource Directory of Scientists and Engineers with Disabilities." $10.00 plus $3.00 shipping and handling.

Rehabilitation Engineering Center of the Smith Kettlewell Eye Research Institute
2232 Webster Street
San Francisco, CA 94115
(415) 561-1619   FAX (415) 561-1610

A federally funded center that develops and tests new technology for individuals who are visually impaired, blind, or deaf-blind, with special projects devoted to computers.

Rehabilitation Technology Association (RTA)
West Virginia Research And Training Center
1 Dunbar Plaza, Suite E
Dunbar, WV 25064-3098
(304) 766-7138   (304) 348-6340 (V/TT)   FAX (304) 766-7846

A membership group of rehabilitation professionals interested in advancing the use of technology by people with disabilities. Operates Project Enable, a computer bulletin board system, with information about disabilities for consumers and professionals. FREE manual. Publishes newsletter, "On Line," available in standard print, audiocassette, and IBM diskette.

Trace Research and Development Center on Communication, Control and Computer Access for Handicapped Individuals
University of Wisconsin - Madison
S-151 Waisman Center, 1500 Highland Avenue
Madison, WI 53705-2280
(608) 263-2309   (608) 263-5408 (TT)   FAX (608) 262-8848

Conducts basic research and product development which have the goal of improving communications and computer access for people with disabilities. Information dissemination, conferences, and training also available.

PROFESSIONAL PUBLICATIONS

Technology and Disability, Andover Medical Publishers, 80 Montvale Avenue, Stoneham, MA 02180

Technology Related Bibliography Update, American Printing House for the Blind, PO Box 6085, Louisville, KY 40206-0085, available on 3 1/2" disks formatted for Apple II computers

Trace Resource Book Assistive Technologies for Communication, Control and Computer Access, Trace Research and Development Center, University of Wisconsin - Madison, S-151 Waisman Center, 1500 Highland Avenue, Madison, WI 53705

Case vignette

Melissa Agronski: Using High Tech Aids to Adjust to Vision Loss

Melissa Agronski is a 30 year old woman who is legally blind due to diabetic retinopathy. More than a year ago, the depression that has accompanied her fluctuating vision caused Ms Agronski to resign from her job as an elementary school teacher. Ms Agronski's ophthalmologist and diabetologist recently had a meeting to discuss her status, including the fact that she seemed to have become extremely withdrawn. They registered her with the state agency that serves individuals who are visually impaired or blind, with a complete report on her physical and psychological condition. Unfortunately, they failed to tell Ms Agronski that she was registered with the state agency. When she received a notice in the mail that she would be receiving a visit from a social worker, her depression turned to anger toward her physicians.

When the state social worker phoned to set up an appointment, Ms Agronski exploded in anger, insisting that she had no need from services from "intrusive strangers who knew nothing about me." The social worker, Maria Hartman, explained that there were many services that could help Ms Agronski, but she would not hear of it. She slammed down the telephone receiver in anger.

Shortly thereafter, a good friend, Tim Broadhurst, paid a visit. Tim was one of the few people who had maintained contact with Melissa during this crisis period. Melissa told Tim about her encounter with Maria Hartman and how angry she was about it. Tim agreed that it was wrong for the physicians to register Melissa without telling her; however, he suggested that she needed to do something about the deteriorating condition of her life and that she give Ms Hartman the opportunity to describe the services she could provide. Ms Agronski was in a calmer and more receptive mood than when she had talked with Ms Hartman and agreed with Tim's suggestion to give her at least one chance. The next day she phoned to set up an appointment.

Maria Hartman turned out to be very different than what Ms Agronski had expected. About the same age as Ms Agronski, Ms Hartman was visually impaired from multiple sclerosis, a condition which also causes fluctuating vision. She described to Ms Agronski her own reactions to vision loss and how she had

Continued on next page

180

also become angry at service providers. On a positive note, she told Ms Agronski about a group that was forming at the local hospital to help people with diabetes and vision loss cope with daily living, emotional responses, and the need to support themselves financially. Led by a nurse who had special training as a diabetes educator, the group required only that participants agree to attend all six initial sessions at the hospital and pay a minimal fee of ten dollars per session. After that time participants could decide whether to continue with additional group sessions or request referrals for specialized services.

Much to her own surprise, Ms Agronski agreed to enroll in the group, where she found several of the participants to be about her age and encountering similar problems. With the help of Jan Abernathy, the nurse who was running the group, Ms Agronski learned about special syringes and glucose monitors with speech output that could help her monitor her diabetes. She also learned that her emotional reactions, which seemed to go to extremes, could have been caused by her inability to control her blood sugar properly. The group members discussed the difficulties in adjusting to vision that is poor one day, worse the next, and improved the following day. It was a relief to hear that her own reactions were not abnormal and that she was not crazy.

The group helped Ms Agronski cope with her emotions and the management of her diabetes, both of which contributed to feeling better about herself. But she still was unemployed and worried about what would happen when her savings ran out. She asked Ms Abernathy to refer her to an organization that could help her realistically assess her employment skills. Ms Abernathy suggested a private rehabilitation consultant who specialized in job placement for people with disabilities. Ms Agronski was concerned about the fee charged by this consultant, but Ms Abernathy assured her that her disability insurance would cover the cost.

Kim Greenbaum, the consultant recommended by Ms Abernathy, was able to see Ms Agronski the following week. Her confidence bolstered, Ms Agronski took public transportation to Ms Greenbaum's office. When Ms Greenbaum asked Ms Agronski what type of work she would like to do, she replied that she had really enjoyed teaching and would like to return. Ms Greenbaum arranged for several vendors of adaptive equipment to come to her office so that they could jointly

Continued on next page

evaluate different types of equipment that would enable Ms Agronski to prepare her lessons and complete reports. After trying several different types of equipment, Ms Agronski decided that she felt most comfortable with a scanner with speech output. This equipment would enable her to read texts and administrative paperwork. Ms Greenbaum suggested that she apply for financial assistance for purchasing this equipment from the state agency. She contacted Ms Hartman to arrange to apply for this funding.

Following receipt of approval for purchasing this equipment, Ms Agronski set up an appointment with the principal of the school where she had previously worked to see if a position was available. Much to her surprise, she learned that her previous position had been filled with a substitute teacher and that she could apply for the position.

Ms Hartman sent reports to the ophthalmologist, diabetologist, nurse, and vocational specialist about Ms Agronski's progress. She suggested that they hold a joint meeting with Ms Agronski in the event that her vision deteriorates further, so that a coordinated plan of rehabilitation could be developed. She also suggested that in the future, the diabetologist and the ophthalmologist inform patients prior to registering them with the state agency.

An Individualized Written Rehabilitation Plan (IWRP) may require that state vocational rehabilitation agencies purchase adaptive equipment and provide training in the use of this equipment. Some states provide full funding; others provide partial funding. Vocational rehabilitation services may also provide job referrals upon completion of training. In some cases, employers may pay for adaptive technology. Community-based service organizations such as Lions Clubs may assist individuals in the purchase of adaptive equipment.

Adaptive equipment may be covered by an insurance settlement, if an insurance company is paying for the patient/client's rehabilitation. The Social Security Administration's PASS Program allows participants to set aside income to obtain funding for assistive equipment. The Social Security Administration will provide information about this program [(800) 772-1213 or (800) 325-0778 (TT)].

REFERRAL RESOURCES

Electronic Industries Foundation (EIF)
919 18th Street, Suite 900
Washington, DC 20006
(202) 955-5810   (202) 955-5836 (TT)

Produces a variety of publications which enable professionals to guide people with disabilities to sources of funding for adaptive equipment.

Financial Aid for Students with Disabilities
HEATH Resource Center
One Dupont Circle, NW
Washington, DC 20036-1193
(800) 544-3284

Includes information about funding assistive technology. Single copy FREE in print and audiocassette; send a blank 3 1/2" or 5 1/4" double density, double sided diskette and indicate choice of MS-DOS compatible or Macintosh.

Financing Adaptive Technology: A Guide to Sources and Strategies for Blind and Visually Impaired Users
by Stephen Mendelsohn
Smiling Interface
PO Box 2792, Church Street Station
New York, NY 10008-2792
(212) 222-0312

Describes federal, state, local and private resources. LARGE PRINT, braille, four-track audiocassette, or Apple or IBM PC disk. $23.00.

Tax Information for Handicapped and Disabled Individuals
Internal Revenue Service, Publication #907
(800) 829-3676   (800) 829-4059 (TT)

Includes information on taxable and nontaxable income items. The cost of adaptive equipment may be deductible. Published annually.

SOURCES OF HIGH TECH AIDS

Closed Circuit Television Systems

Closed Circuit Television Systems (CCTV's) are designed to magnify printed material electronically. The components are a mounted camera, a self-contained light source, a lens that magnifies print to various sizes or one fixed to the individual's specifications, and a monitor. Some models may be used to magnify the screen output of computers.

Humanware, Inc.
6245 King Road
Loomis, CA 95650
(800) 722-3393   (916) 652-7253   FAX (916) 652-7296

Produces the ClearView, with 12 or 17 inch black and white or color desktop monitor, and the Viewpoint, which uses a hand held camera to scan material and transmit it to the monitor.

Optelec
6 Lyberty Way, PO Box 729
Westford, MA 01886
(800) 828-1056   In MA, (508) 392-0707   FAX (508) 692-6073

Produces a variety of models, with 14 or 20 inch monitors. Black and white or color options. Magnification of 8X to 60X depending upon model.

Opteq
Tojek & Associates
17355 Mierow Lane
Brookfield, WI 53005
(414) 784-4979   FAX (414) 784-4478

Models offer options such as split screen, color monitor, and computer access. 13 to 19 inch monitors available.

Seeing Technologies, Inc.
7074 Brooklyn Boulevard
Minneapolis, MN 55429
(800) 462-3738   In MN, (612) 560-8080   FAX (612) 560-0663

Offers a choice of screen sizes and color or black and white monitors.

<u>Telesensory</u>
455 North Bernardo Avenue, PO Box 7455
Mountain View, CA 94039-7455
(800) 227-8418   (415) 960-0920   FAX (415) 969-9064

Produces a variety of monitor sizes, including 14 inch, 19 inch, and hand held models and a choice of colors. Demonstration video, "See for Yourself," FREE. Newsletter, "Focus on Technology," is published three times a year in standard print and audiocassette, FREE.

The options for computer users who have experienced vision loss have increased dramatically over the past few years. Some standard computers on the market are equipped with features that enable users to magnify print size on the screen a specified number of times; for example, the Apple Macintosh includes a standard feature called Close View. Operating systems such as "Windows" also permit the selection of a variety of on screen font sizes when used with an appropriate software program.

Some software packages increase the size of print on the screen of IBM PC's and compatibles and Apple computers. Large monitors may enlarge print size and enable people with vision loss to continue using a standard computer, although they are substantially more expensive than standard size monitors.

Some people with vision loss use synthetic speech screen access, often in conjunction with magnification systems. Speech output reinforces what is displayed on the screen, reduces fatigue, and often allows the use of less magnification and therefore a greater field of view. Pitch, rate, volume, and intonation of the synthetic voice should be considered when choosing a particular speech synthesizer. Optical character readers scan printed text; when used with an adapted computer, this text may be transcribed to speech or braille output.

It is always a good idea to provide headphones to workers who use computers with speech output to avoid disturbing co-workers. Printer hoods may reduce the noise levels of printers that produce braille output.

Organizations

(In the listings below, telephone numbers have symbols V for voice and TT for text telephone where organizations have published this information.)

Access Unlimited-Speech Enterprises
3535 Briarpark Drive, Suite 102
Houston, TX 77042
(800) 848-0311   (713) 461-0006

An information center for special computer resources and products. Over 300 special products are listed in a catalogue available for a $5.00 contribution.

American Printing House for the Blind (APH)
APH Microcomputer Division
1839 Frankfort Avenue, PO Box 6085
Louisville, KY 40206-0085
(800) 223-1839   (502) 895-2405   FAX (502) 895-1509

Sells adaptive computer hardware and software and computer manuals for Apple products in LARGE PRINT, audiocassette, and braille. Publishes newsletter, "Micro Materials Update," in LARGE PRINT and audiocassette, FREE.

Apple Computer, Inc.
Office of Special Education Programs
20525 Mariani Avenue
Cupertino, CA 95014
(408) 996-1010

Offers a packet of information which describes accessibility features for users of Macintosh and Apple II equipment.   FREE

Canadian National Institute for the Blind (CNIB)
Technical Aids Service
1931 Bayview Avenue
Toronto, Ontario M4G 4C8 Canada
(416) 486-2636   FAX (416) 480-7677

Provides consultation and demonstration of high and low tech products and facilitates funding for purchase and maintenance of equipment.

Center for Special Education Technology
Council for Exceptional Children
1920 Association Drive
Reston, VA 22091-1589
(703) 620-3660 (V/TT)   FAX (703) 264-9494

Collects and exchanges information about the use of technology in the education of children and youth with disabilities.

GTE Education Services, Inc.
PO Box 619810
Dallas, TX 75261-9810
(800) 927-3000

Maintains databases related to special education and computer bulletin boards to provide parents and professionals access to information exchange, technical assistance, and resources. Set-up fee of $25.00, annual subscription fee of $35.00, and monthly minimum usage fee of $14.00.

IBM Special Needs Information Referral Center
PO Box 2150
Atlanta, GA 30301-2150
(800) 426-2133   (800) 284-9482 (TT)   In GA, (404) 238-4806

An automated telephone service directs callers through a menu of options such as a list of agencies in their states which can make referrals for technology information and IBM Independence Series products.

National Cristina Foundation
42 Hillcrest Drive
Pelham Manor, NY 10803
(800) 274-7846   (914) 783-7494

Distributes donations of surplus or obsolete computer hardware or software to organizations or individuals with disabilities.

National Easter Seal Society
Computer Assistive Technology Services (CATS)
Technology Related Loan Fund
70 East Lake Street, 9th Floor
Chicago, IL 60601-5907
(312) 726-6200   (312) 726-4258 (TT)   FAX (312) 726-1494

Evaluates and adapts current computer technology for individuals with disabilities. Some Easter Seals affiliates offer CATS programs or serve as information and support centers. Administers grant program for individuals who need financial assistance to purchase assistive technology.

National Technology Center
American Foundation for the Blind (AFB)
15 West 16th Street
New York, NY 10011
(212) 620-2080   FAX (212) 620-2137

Develops and adapts consumer products with speech or tactile output. Evaluations of high tech products conducted by consumers and Center staff are published in "Random Access," a column in the "Journal of Visual Impairment and Blindness" (JVIB). JVIB is available at many university libraries.

Recorded Periodicals
Associated Services for the Blind
919 Walnut Street, 2nd Floor
Philadelphia, PA 19107
(215) 627-0600, extension 208

Subscriptions on four-track audiocassette for popular computer magazines such as "Computers" and "Computerworld," which are not available in special media elsewhere. FREE price list.

Trace Research and Development Center on Communication, Control and Computer Access for Handicapped Individuals
University of Wisconsin-Madison
S-151 Waisman Center
1500 Highland Avenue
Madison, WI 53705-2280
(608) 263-2309   (608) 263-5408 (TT)   FAX (608) 262-8848

Offers workshops in computer access for people with disabilities and a wide variety of publications on computer accessibility. FREE catalogue

Apple Computer Resources in Special Education and Rehabilitation
c/o DLM Teaching Resources
One DLM Park
Allen, TX 75002
(800) 527-4747

A guide that describes more than 1,000 hardware and software products, publications, and organizations. $19.95 plus 9% shipping and handling.

Assistive Technology: A Selective Bibliography
National Library Service for the Blind and Physically Handicapped (NLS)
1291 Taylor Street, NW
Washington, DC 20542
(800) 424-8567 or 8572 (Reference Section)
(800) 424-9100 (to receive application)
(202) 707-5100   FAX (202) 707-0712

Lists books, articles, and pamphlets which describe assistive technology needs, funding sources for technology, periodicals, and information sources. FREE

Closing the Gap
PO Box 68
Henderson, MN 56044
(612) 248-3294   FAX (612) 248-3810

This bimonthly newsletter reviews hardware and software products developed for users with disabilities, U.S., $26.00; Canada and Mexico, $40.00; other countries, $50.00. The organization also provides training and consulting services and holds an annual conference.

Computer-Disability News
National Easter Seal Society
70 East Lake Street, 9th Floor
Chicago, IL 60601-5907
(312) 726-6200   (312) 726-4258 (TT)   FAX (312) 726-1494

Quarterly publication for individuals with disabilities and their families, educators, and rehabilitation professionals. $15.00

Flip Track Learning Systems
2055 Army Trail Road, Suite 100
Addison, IL 60101
(800) 424-8668   FAX (708) 628-0550

Audiocassettes which teach use of software programs such as word processing, spreadsheet, and database management for IBM and compatibles and Macintosh.

The Handbook of Assistive Technology
by Gregory Church and Sharon Glennen
Singular Publishing Group, Inc.
4284 41st Street
San Diego, CA 92015

Provides an overview of funding; adaptive access including LARGE PRINT, speech, and braille. Suggestions for integrating assistive technology in the community and classroom. Product directory. $39.95

Raised Dot Computing Newsletter
Raised Dot Computing, Inc.
408 South Baldwin Street
Madison, WI 53703
(800) 347-9594   (608) 257-9595

This bimonthly newsletter reviews microcomputer applications for users who are visually impaired or blind. U.S., Canada, and Mexico: LARGE PRINT, $18.00; audiocassette, $20.00. FREE sample newsletter available on request. Raised Dot Computing also publishes computer software.

Solutions: Access Technologies for People Who are Blind
by Olga Espinola and Diane Croft
National Braille Press (NBP)
88 St. Stephen Street
Boston, MA 02115
(617) 266-6160   FAX (617) 437-0456

Describes adaptive computer devices, bulletin boards, and publications. Includes interviews with individuals who train others to use adaptive devices. Available in standard print; audiocassette (two, four-track audiocassettes); IBM disk (3 1/2" or 5 1/4"); and braille. U.S., $21.95; Canada, $25.95 (prepaid orders only). Add $3.50 shipping and handling for standard print edition or for UPS shipping, rather than "Free Matter for the Blind."

Technology Update
Sensory Access Foundation
385 Sherman Avenue, Suite 2
Palo Alto, CA 94306
(415) 329-0430   FAX (415) 323-1062

A newsletter that describes recent developments in technology for users who are visually impaired or blind.   Available in standard print, LARGE PRINT, and audiocassette. Individuals in the U.S. who are visually impaired, $30.00, foreign, $47.00; other individuals, U.S., $37.00, foreign, $57.00; organizations, U.S., $47.00, foreign, $67.00.

Computer Center for the Visually Impaired
Baruch College
17 Lexington Avenue, Box 515
New York, NY 10010
(212) 447-3070

Provides training courses in personal computers and software programs; career counseling; and an introductory adaptive computing course for parents and professionals.

Hadley School for the Blind
700 Elm Street
Winnetka, IL 60093
(800) 323-4238   In IL, (708) 446-8111

Offers correspondence courses on microcomputers and word processing for individuals who are legally blind, have a prognosis of legal blindness, or are hearing impaired with a prognosis of visual loss. Requires ability to read at the high school level, FREE. Course catalogue available in LARGE PRINT, audiocassette, and braille. FREE

Lions World Services for the Blind
2811 Fair Park Boulevard
PO Box 4055
Little Rock, AR 72214
(501) 664-7100

Offers courses in computer programming, word processing, and other software packages.

Project CABLE
Carroll Center for the Blind
770 Centre Street
Newton, MA 02158
(617) 969-6200   In MA, (800) 852-3131   FAX (617) 969-6204

Offers evaluation and training in use of LARGE PRINT, speech, and braille output equipment. Tuition fees vary according to eligibility for a variety of subsidy funding sources.

Storer Computer Access Center
Sight Center, Cleveland Society for the Blind
1909 East 101st Street
Cleveland, OH 44106
(216) 791-8118

Evaluation and training center for use of LARGE PRINT, speech, and braille computer access devices. Short term rental of equipment.

University of New Orleans Training and Resource Center for the Blind
ADC 40, Lakefront-East Campus
New Orleans, LA 70148
(504) 286-7096

Academic year and summer continuing education courses in word processing, data base management, medical transcription, and Lotus. Career counseling available.

Arkenstone
1185-D Bordeaux Drive
Sunnyvale, CA 94089
(800) 444-4443   (415) 752-2200   FAX (408) 745-6739

Produces the Arkenstone Reader, a document scanner and character recognition board, which provides speech output from print for IBM PC or compatibles. Available in versions that read English, French, and German. The Ready To Read PC is a portable personal computer compatible with DOS-based hardware and software. An Open Book, designed for individuals without personal computer skills, scans text and converts it to speech. Special prices for individuals who are visually impaired or blind.

Blazie Engineering
109 East Jarrettsville Road, Unit D
Forest Hill, MD 21050
(410) 893-9333   FAX (410) 836-5040

Produces the Braille 'n Speak, a portable talking braille notetaker, which has additional features such as a talking clock and calendar, calculator, and stopwatch. May be used with a computer terminal and a modem. Battery powered speech synthesizer.

DECtalk
Digital Equipment Corporation
Two Penn Plaza
New York, NY 10121
(212) 856-3100

Text-to-speech system converts standard ASCII text to a human quality voice. The speech type and rate are adjustable. Special prices for individuals who are visually impaired or blind.

GW Micro
310 Racquet Drive
Fort Wayne, IN 46825
(219) 483-3625

Produces Sounding Board, an internal speech synthesizer for PC compatible computers. LARGE PRINT, audiocassette, and disk instruction manuals available. Also sells other computer systems, synthesizers, software, and accessories.

Humanware, Inc.
6245 King Road
Loomis, CA 95650
(916) 652-7253   FAX (916) 652-7296

Produces computers with LARGE PRINT, synthetic speech, or braille output; Speakwriter, a talking typewriter; and other adaptive devices.

IBM Personal System/2 Screen Reader
PO Box 2150
Atlanta, GA 30301-2150
(800) 426-2133   (800) 284-9482 (TT)   In GA, (404) 238-4806

Provides speech output of screen text. Compatible with software such as dBase III Plus, Lotus 1-2-3, and DisplayWrite 4.

Mentor O & O Inc.
3000 Longwater Drive
Norwell, MA 02061-1672
(800) 992-7557   (617) 871-6950   FAX (617) 871-7785

Sells the Horizon Low Vision Magnifier, a digital scanner that converts text to a single line which scrolls across a 14 inch monitor. Up to 35X magnification.

Telesensory
455 North Bernardo Avenue, PO Box 7455
Mountain View, CA 94039-7455
(800) 227-8418   (415) 960-0920   FAX (415) 969-9064

Produces LARGE PRINT and speech hardware and software; an optical scanner, designed to be used with LARGE PRINT, speech, and braille systems; and many computer products for people who use braille.

Xerox Imaging Systems/Kurzweil
9 Centennial Park
Peabody, MA 01960
(800) 343-0311   (508) 977-2000

The Xerox/Kurzweil Reader produces speech output from print and from a computer terminal. The portable Kurzweil Personal Reader weighs only 19 pounds.

Ai Squared
PO Box 669
Manchester Center, VT 05255-0669
(802) 362-3612   FAX (802) 362-1670

Produces ZoomText, LARGE PRINT software for IBM compatibles with graphics magnification, Microsoft Windows interface, and font editor. $595.00. inFocus is a memory resident program with 2X magnification for text and graphics. $149.00

Artic Technologies
55 Park Street, Suite 2
Troy, MI 48083-2753
(313) 588-7370   FAX (313) 588-2650

Produces speech synthesizers and screen access systems including hardware, software, tutorials, and accessories. "Visions Newsletter" published three times a year.

Berkeley Systems, Inc.
2095 Rose Street
Berkeley, CA 94709
(510) 540-5535

inLARGE magnifies Macintosh text and graphics, $95.00; outSPOKEN uses the Macintosh's built in speech synthesizer to make word processing programs, spreadsheets, and databases accessible to users who are visually impaired or blind. $395.00

Eye Relief
Ski Soft Publishing
1644 Massachusetts Avenue
Lexington, MA 02173
(800) 662-3622   (617) 863-1876

Designed for IBM PC's and compatibles, this word processing program offers six sizes of on-screen type, oversized cursor, wordwrap scrolling, and LARGE PRINT manual. $295.00

GW Micro
310 Racquet Drive
Fort Wayne, IN 46825
(219) 483-3625

Produces Vocal-Eyes, a screen review reader to be used in conjunction with speech synthesizer. LARGE PRINT, audiocassette, and disk instruction manuals available. $495.00

Humanware, Inc.
6245 King Road
Loomis, CA 95650
(800) 722-3393   (916) 652-7253   FAX (916) 652-7296

Keynote GOLD speech synthesizer with MasterTouch screen reading software, $1875.00. Available in English, French and Spanish.

JAWS (Job Access With Speech)
Henter-Joyce
10901-C Roosevelt Boulevard, Suite 1200
St. Petersburg, FL 33716-2315
(800) 336-5658   (813) 576-5658   FAX (813) 577-0099

A screen access software program to use with a variety of speech synthesizers designed for IBM PC's, IBM PS/2, and compatibles. $495.00 (speech synthesizer not included). Also sells instructional tapes for using WordPerfect and DOS with JAWS.

Kidsview Software, Inc.
PO Box 98
Warner, NH 03278
(800) 542-7501   (603) 927-4428

Specializes in LARGE PRINT software for Apple II, PC/MS-DOS, and Commodore 64 computers. Also sells Kidsword, a LARGE PRINT word processor.

LP DOS
Optelec
6 Lyberty Way, PO Box 729
Westford, MA 01886
(800) 828-1056   In MA, (508) 392-0707   FAX (508) 692-6073

LARGE PRINT software which operates on any IBM or compatible computer. Compatible with speech packages, enabling the user to have speech back-up while using LARGE PRINT software. $495.00. LP-DOS Version 5.0 supports Microsoft Windows. $595.00

Microsystems Software, Inc.
600 Worcester Road
Framingham, MA 01701
(508) 626-8511   FAX (508) 626-8515

Produces MAGic, 2X screen magnification software for DOS and Windows, $79.00, and MAGic Deluxe, up to 12X magnification, $195.00. LARGE PRINT or audiocassette user guide available for MAGic Deluxe. Demonstration copy of MAGic Deluxe available by downloading from the Microsystems Software bulletin board, (508) 875-8009.

ZoomText
Ai Squared
PO Box 669
Manchester Center, VT 05255-0669
(802) 362-3612   FAX (802) 362-1670

A magnification program for IBM PC's and compatibles. Scrolling, viewing and tracking systems, and split screens offer access to word processing programs, data bases, spreadsheets, and communications programs. $495.00

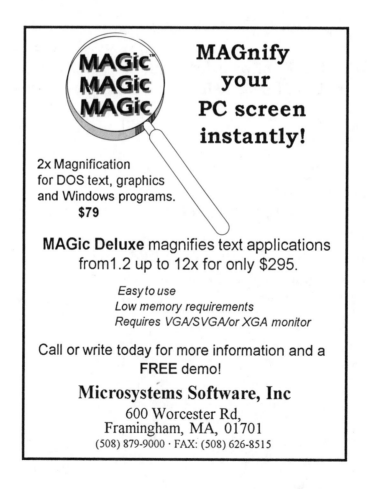

Contrast enhancement filters attach to the computer monitor, increase contrast, and reduce glare from natural and overhead light sources. Visor-like hoods will also shield the monitor from overhead lighting. Local computer supply stores are the best source.

Asymmetric lighting illuminates the work area without glare. Asymmetric lighting is available in desk top models, on flexible arms which may be surface or wall mounted or used with a floor stand. Glare may also be reduced by removing a light bulb or two from an overhead fixture and using a desk lamp to focus on work material. Louvers are available for some lamps to further reduce glare.

Compu-Lenz, which fits on most computer monitors, enlarges character size while eliminating distortion and light reflection. Available from Florida New Concepts Marketing, PO Box 261, Port Richey, FL 34673-0261, (800) 456-7097

Enlarged keyboard labels double the size of letters from standard 18 point to 38 point size and numbers to 32 point. Black print on ivory or white print on black. Braille keytop labels and home-row indicators are also available. Order from Hooleon Corporation, PO Box 230, Department CA92, Cornville, AZ 86325, (602) 634-7515

Typing stands or document holders placed beside or attached to the computer or monitor reduce head and neck movement. Document holders which have flexible arms allow the computer user to move material closer, a useful feature for individuals using low vision aids.

Low-Vision Word Processor:

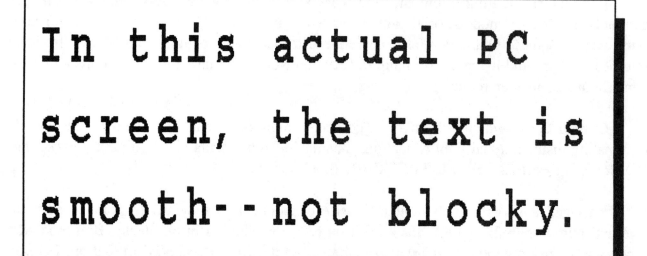 just $295!

In this actual PC screen, the text is smooth--not blocky.

- *Eye Relief* is an award-winning Word Processing program for Low-Vision users. It lets the Low-Vision user do word processing with high-quality screen fonts and complete control over on-screen spacing. *Eye Relief* runs on any PC that has 512K of RAM and a graphics screen. (CGA, EGA, VGA, or Hercules.)

- *Eye Relief* screen fonts can be 1,2,3,4 or 5x normal size--up to 1.4" high on a standard PC screen! As you type and edit, your text will appear in large type--as will on-screen help, pull-down menus, and other messages. Even the *User Guide* is set in 18-point Large Type!

- *Eye Relief* lets you create, edit, and print standard ASCII text files. (This insures compatibility with other word processors, as files created by *Eye Relief* may be loaded easily into WordPerfect, Microsoft Word, and other word processors.)

- Editing functions include Insert, Delete, Cut, Paste, Copy, Find and Replace. Text *wordwraps* at the edge of the screen, so you always see a continuous stream of text. (No need for horizontal scrolling!)

Note: The text shown above would be **TWICE** as large on a standard 14" PC screen.

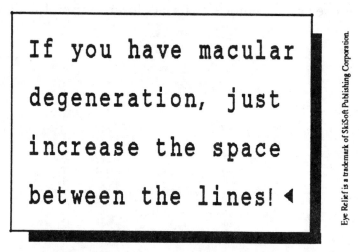

If you have macular degeneration, just increase the space between the lines! ◀

- It prints normal-sized text on any printer, using any margins, headers, footers, and page numbers. It can print 18-point Type on a Laserjet or Postscript printer.

Eye Relief is a product of SkiSoft Publishing Corporation 1644 Massachusetts Ave. Suite 79 Lexington, MA 02173

617-863-1876 Fax: 617-861-0086

Order now--or request a demo!

"Best Special Needs Software of the Year"

Software Publishers Association *Excellence in Software Awards*, Spring 1990

Chapter 7

SPECIAL READING RESOURCES AND SERVICES

People with vision loss frequently cite inability to read as their major complaint. With the many products on the market, reduced vision need not stop individuals from reading. A wide variety of assistive devices and reading material in special media helps people who have experienced vision loss to continue reading books and other materials.

Many individuals use magnifiers, closed circuit television reading systems, or reading machines with speech output. In many communities, agencies provide volunteer readers for people who are visually impaired or blind. The state agency that serves people who are visually impaired or blind or the local United Way office can direct individuals to volunteer reading services in the area.

Special services for people with vision loss and other disabilities are available at many public libraries. Libraries often have closed circuit television reading systems, specially adapted computer equipment, and collections of LARGE PRINT books and books on audiocassette. Portable versions of adapted equipment are available on loan to patrons at some libraries. Many libraries have special outreach or home-bound programs that deliver books to patrons who are unable to get to the library. The reference librarian can describe the services available for people with vision loss.

In the U.S., if an individual is unable to read standard print because of vision loss or physical disability, he or she is eligible for services from the National Library Service for the Blind and Physically Handicapped (See "PROFESSIONAL ORGANIZATIONS" section below). The NLS provides services to people with vision loss, physical limitations which prevent them from holding a book or turning the pages, and those with perceptual problems. A health care or rehabilitation professional must fill out an application that indicates the nature of the disability. Professionals may obtain NLS applications to keep on hand directly from the NLS, from the regional branch of the NLS, or from the state agency that serves individuals who are visually impaired or blind.

In Canada, special library services for individuals who are blind or visually impaired are provided by the Canadian National Institute for the Blind (CNIB), National Library Division, (See "PROFESSIONAL ORGANIZATIONS" section below). CNIB provides audiocassette books and magazines, recorded in English and French, to individuals who are visually impaired or blind. (See "Appendix B: Division Offices of the Canadian National Institute for the Blind.")

Rehabilitation Resource Manual: *VISION Lexington, MA:* *Resources for Rehabilitation copyright 1993*

Service providers should display in their offices a sample of LARGE PRINT books and periodicals, recordings from the National Library Service, and assistive devices. Professionals should be familiar with the services provided by the local public library, and if possible, obtain brochures on their services to distribute to patients or clients. Sometimes a sales representative from a company that manufactures closed circuit televisions or computer equipment with enlarged print or voice output will provide equipment on loan for demonstration to patients or clients or will demonstrate the equipment at a self-help group meeting.

Designed for distribution by professionals, "How to Keep Reading with Vision Loss" is a LARGE PRINT (18 point bold type) publication that describes a variety of alternatives to standard print. Available from Resources for Rehabilitation, 33 Bedford Street, Suite 19A, Lexington, MA 02173. (617) 862-6455 Minimum purchase, 25 copies. $1.75 per copy. Discounts available for purchases of 100 or more copies. See order form on last page of this book.

Case vignette

Bill Fellows: Reading with Vision Loss

Bill Fellows recently retired from a long career as a stockbroker and was looking forward to pursuing his hobbies, fishing and gardening, and continuing to follow his investments. However, the glaucoma that was diagnosed some years ago has recently caused his vision to deteriorate further; he can no longer read the newspaper financial pages or see well enough to tie the complicated flies he uses for fishing.

A visit to Dr. Samuel Robers, his ophthalmologist, confirmed the deterioration of his vision. Neither additional medication nor filtration surgery was able to halt the progression of his vision loss. Dr. Robers completed a certificate of legal blindness in order to register Mr. Fellows with the state agency that serves individuals who are visually impaired or blind. He explained to Mr. Fellows, who had never heard of the state agency, the variety of services that are offered, including volunteer readers, talking books, rehabilitation teaching, and orientation and mobility instruction. Although at first Mr. Fellows was hesitant to "take services" from a state agency, Dr. Robers explained that all citizens who are legally blind are entitled to them. He also told Mr. Fellows about several other patients who had received these services and as a result, they were able to continue with the activities that they found rewarding. He told Mr. Fellows to expect a call from a social worker in about three weeks to set up a home visit that would determine the types of services that would help Mr. Fellows in his daily activities.

Just as Dr. Robers had stated, the social worker, John Haworth, phoned to set up an appointment. He had received a report from Dr. Robers, so he knew that Mr. Fellows had a very restricted field of vision and decreased acuity.   Mr. Haworth asked Mr. Fellows about the activities that were causing difficulty. He suggested that Mr. Fellows might find it useful to join a self-help group of people his age who had also recently experienced vision loss. Mr. Fellows said that he would feel more comfortable joining a group once he had begun to regain some of the skills required for the everyday activities that he enjoyed.

Continued on next page

Fortunately, the public library in the city where Mr. Fellows lives has a center where patrons with vision loss may use specially adapted computer equipment that enables them to keep reading. Mr. Haworth suggested that specially trained librarians could help Mr. Fellows locate appropriate equipment. Mr. Haworth also told Mr. Fellows about the "Talking Books" program available from the National Library Services for the Blind and Physically Handicapped. When Mr. Fellows heard that his favorite financial magazines, "Fortune" and "Money," are available on discs playable on a special "Talking Book" machine, his enthusiasm began to grow. He asked Mr. Haworth how long it would take to receive his equipment and the first issues of these magazines.

At the library, Mr. Fellows discovered that closed circuit televisions enabled him to read the small print of the financial pages, although slowly and with great patience, and that he could even tie one of his "flies" using the same piece of equipment. Encouraged by this initial success, Mr. Fellows phoned Mr. Haworth in order to begin the orientation and mobility lessons and to learn more about joining a self-help group. Mr. Haworth scheduled an appointment with Mr. Fellows and wrote an interim progress report to Dr. Robers.

(In the listings below, telephone numbers have symbols V for voice and TT for text telephone where organizations have published this information.)

Association of Specialized and Cooperative Library Agencies (ASCLA)
American Library Association
50 East Huron Street
Chicago, IL 60611
(800) 545-2433   (312) 944-6780

ASCLA members include librarians who serve individuals who are blind, visually impaired, physically handicapped, deaf, and hearing impaired as well as elders. Publishes newsletter, "Interface."

Canadian National Institute for the Blind Library Division (CNIB)
1929 Bayview Avenue
Toronto, Ontario, M4G 3E8 Canada
(416) 480-7520   FAX (416) 480-7677

CNIB provides audiocassette books and magazines, recorded in English and French, to individuals who are visually impaired or blind.

National Library Service for the Blind and Physically Handicapped
1291 Taylor Street, NW
Washington, DC 20542
(800) 424-8567 or 8572 (Reference Section)
(202) 707-5100   FAX (202) 707-0712

Produces "Reference Circulars," which provide information on special topics; "Subject Bibliographies," which list recorded and braille books; "Reference Bibliographies," which are print publications on special topics; as well as general information brochures and directories. Publishes newsletter, "News," quarterly, FREE.

National Library Service for the Blind and Physically Handicapped (NLS)

1991 <u>Library Resources for the Blind and Physically Handicapped: A Directory with FY 1990 Statistics on Readership, Circulation, Budget, Staff, and Collections</u>

1990 <u>Building a Library Collection on Blindness and Physical Handicaps: Basic Materials and Resources</u>

1989 <u>Library and Information Services to Persons With Disabilities</u>
all available from: National Library Service for the Blind and Physically Handicapped, 1291 Taylor Street, NW, Washington, DC 20542

Recording for the Blind (RFB)
"RFB NEWS For Professionals Working With People With Disabilities" Recording for the Blind, 20 Roszel Road, Princeton, NJ 08540

Velleman, Ruth

1990 <u>Meeting the Needs of People with Disabilities: A Guide for Librarians, Educators and Other Service Professionals</u> Phoenix, AZ: Oryx Press

LARGE PRINT Books

LARGE PRINT books are usually printed in 14 point type or larger. 14 point type is more than twice the size of standard newsprint.

This is a sample of 14 point type.

This is a sample of 16 point type.

This is a sample of 18 point type.

This is a sample of 18 point bold type.

The local public library is the best source for LARGE PRINT books. The "Complete Directory of Large Print Books and Serials," published annually, lists all titles available in LARGE PRINT and should be available in the library's reference section. (Available from Reed Reference Publishing, PO Box 31, New Providence, NJ 07974; $129.95.) Most libraries will arrange interlibrary loans of books they do not own.

LARGE PRINT books are also available for purchase. LARGE PRINT cookbooks, bibles, and reference books are books that readers often want to own rather than borrow. LARGE PRINT books are available in stores and directly from the publishers.

Sources of LARGE PRINT Books

Bolinda Press
PO Box 14402
Shawnee Mission, KS 66285
(800) 848-8810   FAX (913) 894-5526

Hardcover and paperback titles for adults and children. FREE catalogue.

Chivers North America
PO Box 1450
Hampton, NH 03842-0015
(800) 621-0182   (603) 926-8744   FAX (603) 929-3890

Fiction paperback titles, 18 point type. FREE catalogue.

Doubleday Large Print Home Library
6550 East 30th Street
PO Box 6325
Indianapolis, IN 46206-6325
(800) 688-4442   (317) 541-8920

Hardcover popular fiction and nonfiction in LARGE PRINT, priced the same as standard print books. Minimum number of purchases required. FREE catalogue.

G.K. Hall
Order Dept.
100 Front Street, Box 500
Riverside, NJ 08075-7500
(800) 257-5755

Popular fiction and nonfiction titles, 18 point type. Also dictionary, thesaurus, and cookbooks. FREE catalogue.

Grey Castle Press
Pocket Knife Square
Lakeville, CT 06039
(203) 435-2518   FAX (203) 435-8093

Reference books and books for children and adolescents. LARGE PRINT edition of "Consumer Reports" annual buying guide, 14 point type, $29.95. FREE catalogue.

ISIS Large Print Books
Transaction Publishers
Rutgers - The State University of New Jersey
New Brunswick, NJ 08903
(908) 932-2280   FAX (908) 932-3138

Classic and contemporary literature, self-help, and reference books. FREE catalogue.

Random House
400 Hahn Road
PO Box 100
Westminster, MD 21157
(800) 733-3000

Fiction and nonfiction titles, 16 point type. FREE catalogue.

Reader's Digest Large Type Reader
Reader's Digest Fund for the Blind, Inc.
Box 241
Mount Morris, IL 61054-9982
(815) 734-6963

LARGE PRINT selections from Reader's Digest publications, 16 point type. Annual subscription, five volumes; U.S., $9.89; Canada, $12.73.

Reading Materials in Large Type
National Library Service for the Blind and Physically Handicapped (NLS)
1291 Taylor Street, NW
Washington, DC 20542
(800) 424-8567 or 8572 (Reference Section)
(800) 424-9100 (to receive application)
(202) 707-5100   FAX (202) 707-0712

Lists sources of LARGE PRINT reference books, cookbooks, music, specialty magazines, etc. Some NLS libraries also lend LARGE PRINT books. Each state has its own policy.

Thorndike Press
100 Front Street, Box 500
Riverside, NJ 08075-9951
(800) 257-5755   FAX (800) 562-1272

Popular fiction and nonfiction, 16 point type. FREE catalogue.

Ulverscroft & Charnwood Large Print Books
279 Boston Street
Guilford, CT 06437
(800) 955-9659   (203) 453-2080   FAX (203) 458-9841

Classics, contemporary fiction and nonfiction, 16 point type. FREE catalogue.

Talking Books

"Talking Books" is the term used to describe books recorded for use by individuals who are unable to read standard print because of vision loss, physical limitations which prevent them from holding a book or turning the pages, or perceptual problems. "Talking Book" audiocassettes must be played on a special four-track audiocassette player. "Talking Book" discs are flexible, plastic records which must be played on a special slow speed record player. This equipment is FREE on loan from the National Library Service for the Blind and Physically Handicapped (NLS) in the U.S. or the Canadian National Institute for the Blind in Canada (CNIB). Both organizations produce many of the recorded books in their collections.

Recording for the Blind (RFB)
20 Roszel Road
Princeton, NJ 08540
(800) 221-4792   In NJ, (609) 452-0606   FAX (609) 987-8116

Records educational materials for people who are legally blind or have physical or perceptual disabilities. RFB is a major source of recorded textbooks for college students. Requires certification of disability by a medical or educational professional. Charges a one-time registration fee of $25.00. Sells an adapted two and four-track audiocassette player for use with RFB audiocassettes and/or Talking Books, $165.00 plus $3.00 shipping and handling.

Publishes a catalogue of its recent recordings, "Quarterly Disk Catalog" (QDC), produced on IBM, Apple, or Macintosh computer disk, which lists all additions to the RFB library during the previous quarter and includes a catalogue of the RFB electronic text collection. Subscription, $12.00. Newsletter, "RFB News," available in standard print, audiocassette, and electronic text, FREE. Newsletter, "RFB NEWS," available in standard print, audiocassette, and electronic text. FREE

Volunteers Who Produce Books
National Library Service for the Blind and Physically Handicapped (NLS)
1291 Taylor Street, NW
Washington, DC 10542
(800) 424-8567 or 8572 (Reference Section)
(800) 424-9100 (to receive application)
(202) 707-5100   FAX (202) 707-0712

A directory of volunteer groups and individuals in the U.S. who produce LARGE PRINT, audiocassette, and braille books. FREE

Periodicals

Choice Magazine Listening
PO Box 10
Port Washington, NY 11050
(516) 883-8280

A bimonthly audio anthology of articles from standard print periodicals. Must be played on the NLS "talking book" audiocassette player (see "Talking Books" section, above). FREE

<u>Dialogue</u>
c/o Blindskills, Inc.
Box 5181
Salem, OR 97304
(503) 581-4224

Magazine with articles on employment, technology, and everyday living; includes fiction and poetry by authors who are visually impaired or blind. Published quarterly in LARGE PRINT, four-track audiocassette, and braille. $20.00. Sample copy, $3.00.

<u>Magazines in Special Media</u>
National Library Service for the Blind and Physically Handicapped (NLS)
1291 Taylor Street, NW
Washington, DC 20542
(800) 424-8567 or 8572 (Reference Section)
(800) 424-9100 (to receive application)
(202) 707-5100   FAX (202) 707-0712

This LARGE PRINT booklet lists the magazines that are available in LARGE PRINT (FREE), four-track audiocassette, and disc (playable only on the special four-track NLS players). FREE

<u>Matilda Ziegler Monthly Magazine for the Blind</u>
20 West 17th Street
New York, NY 10011
(212) 242-0263

Magazine available on disc (must be played on the special four-track NLS player) and braille. Articles from current periodicals as well as information of special interest to individuals who are visually impaired or blind. FREE

<u>New York Times Large Type Weekly</u>
Mail Subscriptions
CS Box 9564
Uniondale, NY 11565-9564
(800) 631-2580

Weekly news summary from the "New York Times." Crossword puzzles included. 16 point type. Subscription, 26 weeks, $25.00; 52 weeks, $48.00.

<u>Reader's Digest Large-Type Edition</u>
Reader's Digest Fund for the Blind, Inc.
PO Box 241
Mount Morris, IL 61054-9982
(815) 734-6963

Selected articles from the "Reader's Digest," published monthly. U.S., $8.95; Canada, $11.72.

Recorded Periodicals
Associated Services for the Blind
919 Walnut Street, 2nd Floor
Philadelphia, PA 19107
(215) 627-0600, extension 208

Subscriptions on four-track audiocassette for popular magazines which are not available through the Talking Books Program from the NLS (described above). FREE catalogue.

The World At Large
PO Box 190330
Brooklyn, NY 11219
(800) 285-2743   (718) 972-4000   FAX (718) 972-9400

Weekly LARGE PRINT newspaper with articles reprinted from major news magazines. 52 weeks, U.S., $65.00, Canada, $80.00; 26 weeks, U.S., $37.00, Canada, $47.00. FREE sample available on request.

Electronic Publishing

A recent advance in publishing is the production of publications in electronic format, using computer disks and CD-ROMs, which are similar to musical compact disks. To date, reference works are the most commonly produced works on CD-ROM, although other types of books are coming on the market in this format as well. Since these publications are used with personal computers, they can be accessed by computers that have speech output systems.

Franklin Electronic Publishers, Inc.
122 Burrs Road
Mt. Holly, NJ 08060
(800) 762-5382   (609) 261-4800   FAX (609) 261-2984

Electronic reference publications with speech output, including English and bilingual dictionaries and thesauruses. FREE catalogue.

Recording for the Blind (RFB)
20 Roszel Road
Princeton, NJ 08540
(800) 221-4792   In NJ, (609) 452-0606   FAX (609) 987-8116

E-text, RFB's collection of electronic books on computer disk, includes computer manuals and reference books available for purchase. RFB's catalogue, "Quarterly Disk Catalog" (QDC), produced on IBM, Apple, or Macintosh computer disk, lists all additions (recorded books and E-text) to the RFB library. $12.00. (See "Talking Books" section above for additional information about RFB.)

Commercial Sources of Recorded Materials

Bookstores and libraries now carry recorded books on a variety of subjects. These books do not require special playback equipment (unlike the Talking Books listed above); they may be played on standard audiocassette tape players. Often recorded books are abridged versions of the original books. The companies listed below, however, produce unabridged audiocassettes. "Words on Cassette" (NY: R.R. Bowker), published annually and available at the reference desk of public libraries, lists commercial sources of books recorded on audiocassette.

Bookcassette Sales
1810-B Industrial Drive
PO Box 481
Grand Haven, MI 49417
(800) 222-3225   FAX (800) 648-2312

Bestsellers which must be played on stereo tape players. FREE catalogue.

Books On Tape
PO Box 7900
Newport Beach, CA 92658
(800) 626-3333

Bestsellers available for rent. FREE catalogue.

G.K. Hall
Order Dept.
100 Front Street, Box 500
Riverside, NJ 08075-7500
(800) 257-5755

Bestsellers. FREE catalogue.

Recorded Books
270 Skipjack Road
Prince Frederick, MD 20658
(800) 638-1304

Fiction and nonfiction titles available for rent or purchase. FREE catalogue.

Sterling Audio
100 Front Street, Box 500
Riverside, NJ 08075-9951
(800) 257-5755   FAX (800) 562-1272

Fiction titles. FREE catalogue.

Radio Reading Services

Radio reading services are accessible through special closed channel radio receivers. These services read local newspapers, bestsellers, and special consumer programs. The name and address of a local radio reading service is available from the state agency that provides services to individuals who are visually impaired or blind. Some state agencies provide receivers to eligible clients; some radio reading services will provide FREE receivers.

Religious Materials in Special Media

Bible Alliance, Inc.
PO Box 621
Bradenton, FL 34206
(813) 748-3031   FAX (813) 748-2625

Audiocassettes of the bible and bible studies in English and other languages. Requires certification of visual impairment by the National Library Service for the Blind and Physically Handicapped or similar organization. FREE

Bibles, Other Scriptures, Liturgies and Hymnals in Special Media
National Library Service for the Blind and Physically Handicapped (NLS)
1291 Taylor Street, NW
Washington, DC 20542
(800) 424-8567 or 8572 (Reference Section)
(800) 424-9100 (to receive application)
(202) 707-5100   FAX (202) 707-0712

Reference circular lists religious materials available in special media. Available in standard print and disc (playable on slow speed Talking Book record player). FREE

Christian Record Services
4444 South 52nd Street, Box 6097
Lincoln, NE 68506
(402) 488-0981

Publishes a variety of religious magazines for bible study in LARGE PRINT, audiocassette, and braille. Operates a FREE lending library. FREE catalogue.

Directory of Resources for the Blind and Visually Impaired
John Milton Society for the Blind
475 Riverside Drive, Room 455
New York, NY 10115
(212) 870-3335

LARGE PRINT directory of religious and secular materials in LARGE PRINT, audiocassette, disc, and braille. FREE

Jewish Braille Institute
110 East 30th Street
New York, NY 10016
(212) 889-2525

Loans LARGE PRINT English and Hebrew books. Lending library of recordings in English, Hebrew, Yiddish, and other languages. "JBI Voice" is a monthly audiocassette magazine of Jewish current events and stories. Publishes a LARGE PRINT Jewish calendar. Services are FREE.

Scriptures for Those with Special Needs
American Bible Society
PO Box 5656, Grand Central Station
New York, NY 10164-0851
(212) 408-1499

Lists bibles available in LARGE PRINT as well as audiocassette and braille. Spanish versions available. FREE catalogue.

Walker and Company
720 Fifth Avenue
New York, NY 10019
(800) 289-2553   (212) 265-3632   FAX (212) 307-1764

Religious titles, biographies, fiction, and nonfiction. FREE catalogue.

Chapter 8

ADAPTATIONS FOR PEOPLE WITH VISION LOSS

OPTICAL AIDS

Individuals with vision loss should always be evaluated by a trained professional who conducts a low vision assessment, tries a variety of aids, and allows a trial loan period of aids. Individuals who purchase magnifiers without a professional assessment are unlikely to obtain aids that provide optimal assistance.

The wide variety of optical aids available to people with vision loss may prove to be confusing. It is important that individuals with vision loss understand that not all aids will help with their particular problem and that different aids must be used for different activities. Service providers must be patient in understanding that people with vision loss may be frustrated if the use of an aid does not result in immediate success.

Training in the proper use of an optical aid and perseverance in practicing with the aid will contribute to success. Some individuals will reject aids because they are bulky, hard to handle, or their use attracts undue attention. Service providers should remind people with vision loss that learning to read and do other familiar tasks that once were taken for granted may be very slow at first, but with practice, the results may prove to be rewarding. They should also inform patients or clients that if their vision changes, it may be necessary to be re-evaluated for a new aid.

Researchers and engineers are developing new aids to help individuals with vision loss use their remaining vision to the fullest extent possible. Professionals and service providers should ensure that individuals who use optical or nonoptical low vision aids are informed about new developments.

Corning Medical Optics
MP 21-2-2
Corning, NY 14831
(800) 742-5273   (607) 974-7823

Produces glare control lenses that filter out ultraviolet light and certain short blue wavelengths. Useful for patients who experience photophobia resulting from a variety of conditions.

Designs for Vision
760 Koehler Avenue
Ronkonkoma, NY 11779
(800) 345-4009   (516) 585-3300   FAX (516) 585-3404

Makes a wide variety of optical aids including magnifiers, telescopes, and other optical aids.

Eschenbach Optik of America
904 Ethan Allen Highway
Ridgefield, CT 06877
(203) 438-7471

Makes a wide variety of optical aids including magnifiers, telescopes, and combination lamp/magnifiers.

Keeler
456 Parkway
Broomall, PA 19008
(800) 523-5620   (215) 353-4350   FAX (215) 353-7814

Makes a variety of magnifiers and telescopes.

NoIR
PO Box 159
South Lyon, MI 48178
(800) 521-9746   (313) 769-5565   FAX (313) 769-1708

Makes sunglasses that filter out infrared rays.

NONOPTICAL AIDS

The wide variety of nonoptical aids on the market helps to make everyday living easier for people with vision loss. Many of these aids and devices are used in conjunction with optical aids.

A bold point pen with bold line paper is a simple suggestion for carrying out everyday writing tasks. Writing guides, signature guides, and check writing guides help people to locate lines on a printed page or to line up their own handwritten lines.

Aids that help people carry out their household tasks include assistive devices for the kitchen, such as special cutting devices, markings for stove dials, special measuring and pouring utensils, labels for marking canned goods, and LARGE PRINT cookbooks. Telephones with large numerals or LARGE PRINT dials and LARGE PRINT covers to fit over pushbutton phones are also available. Many appliance manufacturers supply special markers for washing machines, dryers, and other appliances, although it is possible for people to make their own markers at home by using nail polish or other suitable materials.

ENVIRONMENTAL ADAPTATIONS

Although it is not usually necessary to make major structural modifications to enable people with vision loss to function in their home, work, or leisure environment, many factors can contribute to their comfort and safety. Good lighting is essential, along with uncluttered hallways and aisles. The use of contrasting colors for furniture, carpeting, and signs is helpful. Many modern appliances, such as microwave ovens, make independent living easier for people with vision loss.

Health care professionals should make referrals to rehabilitation teachers and occupational therapists, who will visit the home of the person with vision loss, conduct a functional assessment, and assist with environmental adaptations and training. These professionals work in state and private agencies, in private practice, and in hospitals.

(In the listings below, telephone numbers have symbols V for voice and TT for text telephone where organizations have published this information.)

Electronic Industries Foundation (EIF)
919 18th Street, Suite 900
Washington, DC 20006
(202) 955-5810   (202) 955-5836 (TT)

Produces a variety of publications which enable professionals to guide people with disabilities to sources of funding for adaptive equipment.

Rehabilitation Engineering Center of the Smith Kettlewell Eye Research Institute
2232 Webster Street
San Francisco, CA 94115
(415) 567-0667

Develops and tests new technology for individuals who are visually impaired or blind and individuals who are deaf-blind.

PROFESSIONAL PUBLICATIONS

Cocke, Elizabeth A.
1992 "Housing Modifications for Persons Who are Blind or Visually Impaired" RE:view
     XXIV(Spring)1:23-28

Organizations

(In the listings below, telephone numbers have symbols V for voice and TT for text telephone where organizations have published this information.)

ABLEDATA
8455 Colesville Road, Suite 935
Silver Spring, MD 20910-3319
(800) 346-2742   (301) 588-9284

A database of disability-related products for personal care, recreation, and transportation. First 20 items from database search, FREE; a fee is charged for longer searches.

Barrier-Free Design Centre
2075 Bayview Avenue
Toronto, Ontario M4N 3M5 Canada
(416) 480-6000   FAX (416) 480-0009

Provides education, information, and technical consultation in barrier-free design and construction for Canadians with disabilities. Publishes professional guides for barrier-free design. Publishes "The Sourcebook" which provides design recommendations for new construction and residential renovations. $45.00 plus $3.00 shipping, Canadian funds.

Center for Accessible Housing
North Carolina State University
Box 8613
Raleigh, NC 27695-8613
(919) 737-3082 (V/TT)

A federally funded research and training center that works toward improving housing for people with disabilities. Provides technical assistance, training, and publications. Publishes newsletter, "News," available in standard print, LARGE PRINT, audiocassette, and computer disk. FREE

Aids for Everyday Living with Vision Loss
Resources for Rehabilitation
33 Bedford Street, Suite 19A
Lexington, MA 02173
(617) 862-6455   FAX (617) 861-7517

Designed for distribution by professionals, this LARGE PRINT (18 point bold) publication describes major sources of adapted aids for people with vision loss. $1.25 per copy, minimum purchase 25 copies. Discounts for purchases of 100 copies or more. See order form on last page of book.

The Do-Able Renewable Home
by John P. S. Salmen
American Association of Retired Persons (AARP)
Consumer Affairs-Program Department
601 E Street, NW
Washington, DC 20049
(202) 434-2277

Describes how individuals with disabilities can modify their homes for independent living. Room by room modifications are accompanied by illustrations. FREE

Home Safety Checklist for Older Consumers
U.S. Consumer Product Safety Commission
Washington, DC 20207
(800) 638-2772

Provides information on simple, inexpensive repairs and safety recommendations. Single copy, FREE. Available in English and Spanish.

Housing and Support Services for Physically Disabled Persons in Canada
Canadian Rehabilitation Council for the Disabled (CRCD)
45 Sheppard Avenue East, Suite 801
Toronto, Ontario M2N 5W9 Canada
(416) 250-7490 (V/TT)   FAX (416) 229-1371

Lists accessible housing options and other support services for people who live in Canada. $5.00 plus $3.00 shipping and handling, Canadian funds.

Independent Living
Public Affairs Directorate
Health & Welfare Canada
Disabled Persons Unit
Ottawa, Ontario K1A 1B5 Canada

A series of pamphlets on independent living; includes food preparation, appliances, reaching aids, bathroom equipment and bathing aids, and lifting aids. FREE

Making Life More Livable
by Irving R. Dickman
American Foundation for the Blind (AFB)
15 West 16th Street
New York, NY 10011
(800) 232-5463   (212) 620-2000   FAX (212) 620-2105

This LARGE PRINT guide uses pictures to demonstrate many adapted aids. $12.95 plus $3.00 postage and handling. Also available FREE on four-track Talking Book audiocassette from the National Library Service, RC 22319.

Seeing With the Brain
by Mildred Frank
VISION Foundation, Inc.
818 Mt. Auburn Street
Watertown, MA 02172
(617) 926-4232   In MA, (800) 852-3029

This booklet teaches audible and raised letter methods of labeling and filing as well as other helpful techniques. LARGE PRINT and audiocassette, $10.00

Self-Help Publications for Visually Impaired Individuals and Professionals
VISIONS
817 Broadway, 11th floor
New York, NY 10003
(212) 477-3800   FAX (212) 477-6613

Home study kits for self-help rehabilitation include basic indoor mobility, housekeeping skills, personal management, and sensory development. Each kit contains audiocassettes, LARGE PRINT transcript, and performance evaluation criteria. FREE catalogue.

A Street to Share
Foundation Centre Louis-Hebert
525 boulevarde Hamel Est, aile J
Quebec, Quebec G1M 2S8 Canada
(418) 529-6991

This videotape presents typical situations experienced by individuals who are visually impaired or blind as they travel in their community. Makes suggestions for efficient and effective assistance. $25.00 plus $3.00 shipping and handling, U.S. funds.

Tools for Independent Living and Designs for Independent Living
Appliance Information Service (AIS)
Whirlpool Corporation
Administrative Center
Benton Harbor, MI 49022

Provide information on adaptations for major appliances such as control panel overlays, large graphics, and oversized pushbuttons. Also provides use and care manuals and cookbooks in LARGE PRINT, audiocassette, and braille. FREE

Unless otherwise noted, the following vendors offer a range of products, including talking items, magnifiers, kitchen aids, recreational products, and computers. Catalogues are FREE and in standard print, unless otherwise noted.

Access with Ease
PO Box 1150
Chino Valley, AZ 86323
(602) 636-9469

Ann Morris Enterprises
890 Fams Court
East Meadow, NY 11554
(516) 292-9232

Catalogue available in LARGE PRINT, audiocassette, IBM and Apple format disk, FREE. Braille catalogue, $10.00.

AT & T Special Needs Center
2001 Route 46
Parsippany, NJ 07054-1315
(800) 233-1222   (800) 833-3232 (TT)

Provides self-adhesive LARGE PRINT overlays for rotary dial and pushbutton phones, FREE. Sells Big Button Plus Telephone with white numerals on a black background, volume control, and automatic dialing.

Florida New Concepts Marketing
PO Box 261
Port Richey, FL 34673
(800) 456-7097

Sells Beam Scope, which enlarges television picture up to two times, and CompuLenz, which magnifies computer screens. Prices vary with screen size.

Independent Living Aids, Inc. (ILA)
27 East Mall
Plainview, NY 11803
(800) 537-2118   (516) 752-8080

Standard print catalogue. Also available in voice indexed audiocassette for $3.00, which may be applied to an order.

Lighthouse Low Vision Products
36-20 Northern Boulevard
Long Island City, NY 11101
(800) 453-4925   (718) 937-6959   FAX (718) 786-0437

LARGE PRINT catalogue.

LS & S Group
PO Box 673
Northbrook, IL 60065
(800) 468-4789   In IL, (708) 498-9777

Standard print catalogue. Audiocassette catalogue, $3.00, applied to purchase.

Maxi-Aids
42 Executive Boulevard
PO Box 3209
Farmingdale, NY 11735
(800) 522-6294   (516) 752-0521

Standard print catalogue. Audiocassette catalogue, $2.50, refundable as a coupon with purchase of $25.00 or more.

Medic Alert
PO Box 1009
Turlock, CA 95381-1009
(800) 344-3226   In CA, (209) 668-3333

Medical identification bracelet for people with chronic eye conditions and other diseases.

Mons International
6595 Roswell Road, NE, # 224
Atlanta, GA 30329-3152
(800) 541-7903   In Atlanta, (404) 344-8805

Products for People with Vision Problems
American Foundation for the Blind Product Center
PO Box 7044
100 Enterprise Place
Dover, DE 19903-7044
(800) 829-0500

Standard print, audiocassette, and braille catalogues.

Science Products
Box 888
Southeastern, PA 19399
(800) 888-7400   FAX (215) 296-0488

"Vision Aids Resource Guide" offers optical and nonoptical aids. "Technilog" offers specially adapted scientific and technical instruments plus standard aids. "Magnilog" features magnifiers and adaptive aids for everyday living.

Sears Healthcare Catalog
Sears, Roebuck and Co.
PO Box 7003
Downers Grove, IL 60515-8003
(800) 326-1750   (800) 733-4833 (TT)

Offers health care products. Sears HealthCare will file for Medicare reimbursement for customers. In-home or on-site service available.

Sharp Electronics Corporation
Optonica Product Department
PO Box 650
Mahwah, NJ 07430
(201) 529-0322

Manufactures a voice-synthesized VCR (videotape recorder) which gives audible instructions for video recording. Will refer to local distributors.

Shoppers' Guide for Telephone Users with Special Needs
Tele-Consumer Hotline
1910 K Street, NW, Suite 610
Washington, DC 20006
(800) 332-1124 (V/TT)   (202) 223-4371 (V/TT)   FAX (202) 466-6020

LARGE PRINT and braille catalogues.

Vis-Aids
102-09 Jamaica Avenue
PO Box 26
Richmond Hill, NY 11418
(800) 346-9579   (718) 847-4734   FAX (718) 441-2550

<u>Visual Aids and Informational Material</u>
National Association for the Visually Handicapped (NAVH)
22 West 21st Street
New York, NY 10010
(212) 889-3141

LARGE PRINT catalogue.

<u>Worldwide Games</u>
PO Box 517
Colchester, CT 06415-0517
(800) 243-9232   FAX (203) 537-2866

Catalogue of games and crafts.

Chapter 9

LEISURE ACTIVITIES FOR PEOPLE WITH VISION LOSS

Health care and rehabilitation professionals should inquire about the recreational activities and hobbies which the individual with vision loss enjoys. In many cases, this information will enable the professional to motivate people to use optical or nonoptical aids in order to continue a favorite pastime. For example, people who enjoy fishing may continue to tie flies with the use of a stand magnifier or closed circuit television. Crafts enthusiasts use LARGE PRINT patterns, self-threading needles, or hands-free magnifiers to knit, crochet, or cross-stitch. Adapted equipment and special events allow many individuals to participate in sports such as downhill and cross-country skiing, bowling, bicycling, and golf, to name just a few.

Some individuals with vision loss will need assistance in order to continue with these hobbies or sports. Others may develop an interest in a new hobby or sport as a means of socializing with organized groups or individuals. The state agency that serves individuals who are visually impaired or blind can refer individuals to local programs.

PROFESSIONAL ORGANIZATIONS

<u>Center for Recreation and Disability Studies</u>
Curriculum in Leisure Studies and Recreation Administration
CB #8145, 730 Airport Road, Suite 204
University of North Carolina at Chapel Hill
Chapel Hill, NC 27599-8145
(919) 962-0534

Conducts research, training, and demonstration projects. Developed the LIFE Program (Leisure is for Everyone) to train recreation professionals in the community to work with individuals with disabilities; includes a videotape, training guide, resource manual, and support manual. FREE publications list.

CAMPS

Camp programs are available in various locations throughout the U.S. for children and adults who are visually impaired or blind. Some are sponsored by organizations which serve only people who are visually impaired or blind; others offer integrated programs with sighted campers. In addition to traditional summer camp programs, some organizations offer week-long and weekend programs throughout the year. Financial assistance is often available.

Guide to Accredited Camps
American Camping Association (ACA)
Bradford Woods
5000 State Road 67 North
Martinsville, IN 46151
(800) 428-2267

Lists every ACA-accredited camp in the U.S. and includes an index of special programs for campers with disabilities. $10.95

Guide to Summer Camps and Summer Schools
Porter Sargent Publishers, Inc.
11 Beacon Street, Suite 1400
Boston, MA 02108
(617) 523-1670   FAX (617) 523-1021

Lists summer educational and recreation programs including specialized programs for individuals with disabilities. $26.00

CRAFTS

Many individuals with vision loss sew, knit, and crochet and engage in other forms of needlework and crafts. A technique as simple as using light colored knitting needles when knitting with dark colored yarn may enable individuals to continue this hobby. Special tools and guides make it possible for individuals to do woodworking, wallpapering, painting, and an entire range of practical as well as decorative crafts.

Crafts Resources in Special Media
VISION Foundation, Inc.
818 Mt. Auburn Street
Watertown, MA 02172
(617) 926-4232   In MA, (800) 852-3029

A LARGE PRINT list of crafts instruction manuals, kits, and other resources available in LARGE PRINT, audiocassette, and braille. FREE

Many individuals with vision loss wish to continue playing their favorite sports and games. They use adaptive aids or new techniques to compensate for their vision loss. Others find that sports organizations for individuals with disabilities offer them the opportunity to continue familiar recreational pursuits or learn new skills, but with peers who have the same disability. The resources listed below will direct individuals to these organizations.

Sedentary recreational activities such as board games and cards are also accessible to individuals with vision loss. The catalogues listed in Chapter 8, " Adaptations for People with Vision Loss," offer many adapted games such as checkers, chess, Monopoly, crossword puzzles, bingo, and others.

National Library Services for the Blind and Physically Handicapped (NLS)
1291 Taylor Street, NW
Washington, DC 20542
(800) 424-8567 or 8572 (Reference Section)
(800) 424-9100 (to receive application)
(202) 707-5100   FAX (202) 707-0712

"Sports, Outdoor Recreation and Games for Visually and Physically Impaired Individuals" is a reference circular which lists national organizations, literature, and sources for adapted sports equipment and games. FREE. Leisure Pursuit Bibliographies list books available through the NLS on audiocassette, disc, or in braille. Subjects include birding, fishing, horses, sailing, and swimming. The bibliographies are available in LARGE PRINT, disc, or braille. FREE

Popular Activities & Games for Blind, Visually Impaired, & Disabled People
American Foundation for the Blind (AFB)
15 West 16th Street
New York, NY 10011
(800) 232-5463   (212) 620-2000   FAX (212) 620-2105

Lists 50 indoor and outdoor games and activities suitable for individuals of all ages. LARGE PRINT. $12.95 plus $3.00 shipping.

Sharing the Fun: A Guide to Including Persons with Disabilities in Leisure and Recreation
Canadian Rehabilitation Council for the Disabled (CRCD)
45 Sheppard Avenue East, Suite 801
Toronto, Ontario M2N 5W9 Canada
(416) 250-7490 (V/TT)   FAX (416) 229-1371

Provides information on including people with disabilities in leisure activities. $5.95 plus $3.00 shipping and handling, Canadian funds.

Many individuals who experience vision loss wish to continue playing musical instruments, singing, and reading about music. The National Library Service for the Blind and Physically Handicapped (NLS) offers a special music collection through its program of braille and recorded books and magazines. Individuals interested in this program receive materials directly from the NLS in Washington, DC rather than through the network of regional libraries. All materials are mailed to patrons and returned to the NLS postage-free.

NLS Music Services include LARGE PRINT, braille, and recorded scores; musical instruction (for instruments such as guitar, piano, organ, and accordion); and six music magazines, available in a variety of formats. Subscriptions are FREE. Some music publishers produce LARGE PRINT music books; many of these have LARGE PRINT words for familiar songs and hymns without the scores. The NLS Music Service can provide names and addresses of these publishers. Individuals should call the NLS Music Section for specific details, (800) 424-8567.

Individuals with vision loss may find that it is easier to follow the printed score if they use an adjustable music stand which will allow them to bring the music closer to them. Several models are available from the American Printing House for the Blind, 1859 Frankfort Avenue, Louisville, KY 40206. (800) 223-1839 FREE catalogue. Typing stands may also serve as music stands. A weighted base or clamp secures the typing stand to the piano or music stand and the flexible arm allows the score to be moved into view.

SPECIAL MEDIA SERVICES

Descriptive Video Service (DVS) uses an additional channel (SAP) to provide an oral description of a television program's actions and settings. It is accessible through a stereo television, a stereo VCR, or a special stereo attachment to a television. At present, DVS is available on a small portion of public broadcasting's program schedule. Contact your local public broadcasting station to ask if it carries DVS programming. In some areas, the DVS narration is broadcast over the local radio reading service.

Narrative Television Network (NTN) produces talk shows and describes movie classics which are broadcast four hours per week on cable systems nationwide. Free to cable operators and stations, it is available to listeners without additional equipment. The narration is part of the main sound channel, not transmitted on a separate SAP channel. The local cable system can advise individuals if it carries NTN.

Radio reading services, described in Chapter 7, "Special Reading Resources and Services," are sometimes broadcast on cable television stations. The local cable system can advise individuals whether this service is available.

Audiovision
416 Holladay Avenue
San Francisco, CA 94110
(415) 641-4589

Provides descriptive narrative of art exhibits, television, plays, and other media. Provides training to individuals and organizations.

Descriptive Video Service (DVS)
WGBH
125 Western Avenue
Boston, MA 02134
(617) 492-2777, extension 3490

The national DVS broadcast service through which public broadcasting stations receive DVS programs. DVS publishes "DVS Guide," in LARGE PRINT, audiocassette, and braille, FREE. Sells DVS home videotapes; call (800) 736-3099 for a FREE catalogue.

TRAVEL

When planning trips, individuals should inquire about accessibility for people with vision loss at places they plan to visit. The Americans with Disabilities Act requires that public accommodations be accessible to people with disabilities. Public accommodations are broadly defined to include hotels, restaurants, stores, and other sites frequented by travelers. Some museums and historical sites have special tours, literature in LARGE PRINT, or tour guides on audiocassette.

Numerous travel agents and tour operators specialize in arrangements for people with disabilities. Tourist offices and private organizations throughout North America and Europe as well as in many other industrialized countries can provide information about accessibility. LARGE PRINT and/or braille elevator buttons, braille menus, and bathroom safety devices, such as grab bars and nonskid tubs, are examples of these special access features.

Access America: An Atlas and Guide to the National Parks for Visitors with Disabilities
Northern Cartographic
Department BG, PO Box 133
Burlington, VT 05402
(802) 860-2886

Maps of national parks in the U.S. with special features for readers with vision loss. Describes availability of trail guides in LARGE PRINT or braille. $44.95 plus $5.00 shipping and handling.

Access to Art: A Museum Directory for Blind and Visually Impaired People
Museum of American Folk Art Book and Gift Shop
2 Lincoln Square
New York, NY 10023
(212) 977-7298

Lists museums, historical societies, and other facilities that have special services for people with vision loss. Available in LARGE PRINT, audiocassette, and braille. $11.95 plus $3.00 shipping.

CC Inc. Auto Tape Tours
PO Box 227/2 Elbrook Drive
Allendale, NJ 07401
(201) 236-1666

Audiocassettes and videotapes that serve as previews for trips or walking tour guides. FREE catalogue.

Easy Access to National Parks: The Sierra Club Guide for People with Disabilities
by Wendy Roth and Michael Tompane
Sierra Club Books
100 Bush Street, 13th Floor
San Francisco, CA 94104
(415) 291-1600   FAX (415) 291-1602

Reviews accessibility of 50 national parks for individuals with vision, hearing or mobility impairments. $16.00 plus $3.00 shipping and handling. Available in braille from the National Library Service for the Blind and Physically Handicapped, 1291 Taylor Street, NW, Washington, DC 20542.

Hammond Large Type World Atlas
G.K. Hall
Order Dept.
100 Front Street, Box 500
Riverside, NJ 08075-7500
(800) 257-5755

$28.95 plus 10% shipping and handling.

National Park Service
Department of the Interior, Office of Public Affairs
PO Box 37127
Washington, DC 20013-7127

Operates the Golden Access Passport program which admits people who are legally blind or have other disabilities to national parks at no charge and provides a 50% discount on other fees charged by the Park Service. May be obtained at National Parks by providing a certificate of legal blindness. FREE brochure.

Travel Information Center
Moss Rehabilitation Hospital
1200 West Tabor Road
Philadelphia, PA 19141-3099
(215) 456-9600   (215) 456-9602 (TT)

Supplies travel accessibility information about three different locations worldwide for a fee of five dollars.

Travelin' Talk
PO Box 3534
Clarksville, TN 37043-3534
(615) 552-6670   FAX (615) 552-1182

A network of individuals and organizations that provides assistance to travelers with disabilities. Newsletter, "Travelin' Talk," available in LARGE PRINT, audiocassette, and braille; annual contribution requested.

APPENDIX A

STATE AGENCIES FOR INDIVIDUALS WHO ARE VISUALLY IMPAIRED OR BLIND

To learn the address of the state agency nearest you, contact the main office listed below or the information operator for the state government. Toll-free telephone numbers usually operate only within the state.

Alabama
Adult Vocational Rehabilitation and Child Rehabilitation Services
Services for the Deaf and Blind
PO Box 11586
Montgomery, AL 36111-0586
(205) 281-8780 (V/TT)   FAX (205) 281-1973

Alaska
Office of Vocational Rehabilitation
801 West 10th Street, Suite 200
Juneau, AK 99801
(907) 465-2814 (V/TT)   FAX (907) 465-2856

Arizona
State Services for the Blind
4620 North 16th Street
Phoenix, AZ 85016
(800) 255-1850   (602) 255-1850 (V/TT)   FAX (602) 235-9491

Arkansas
Division of Services for the Blind
411 Victory Street, PO Box 3237
Little Rock, AR 72203
(800) 482-5850, extension 324-9270
(501) 324-9281   (501) 324-9271 (TT)   FAX (501) 324-9280

California
Department of Rehabilitation
Services for the Blind and Partially Sighted
830 K Street Mall, Room 222
Sacramento, CA 95814
(916) 445-9040   FAX (916) 327-6919

Colorado
Rehabilitation Center for the Blind and Visually Impaired
2211 West Evans Street
Denver, CO 80223
(303) 937-1226 (V/TT)   FAX (303) 934-6854

Connecticut
Services for the Blind
170 Ridge Road
Wethersfield, CT 06109
(800) 842-4510   (203) 249-8525 (V/TT)   FAX (203) 278-6920

Delaware
Division for the Visually Impaired
1901 North Dupont Highway
Biggs Building
Newcastle, DE 19720
(302) 577-4731   FAX (302) 577-4763

District of Columbia
Visual Impairment Section
Rehabilitation Services Administration
605 G Street, NW, 9th Floor
Washington, DC 20001
(202) 727-0907   (202) 727-0908 (TT)   FAX (202) 727-1707

Florida
Division of Blind Services
Koger Executive Center
2540 Executive Center Circle, West
Tallahassee, FL 32399
(800) 342-1828   (904) 488-1330 (V/TT)   FAX (904) 487-1804

Georgia
Division of Rehabilitation Services
1568 Willingham Drive, Suite F200
College Park, GA 30337
(800) 359-1112   (404) 669-3450 (V/TT)   FAX (404) 669-2922

Guam
Department of Vocational Rehabilitation
122 IT & E Plaza, Room B201
Harmon, Guam 96911
646-9468 (for international calls, dial 671 for country code)

Hawaii
Department of Human Services
Services for the Blind Branch
1901 Bachelot Street
Honolulu, HI 96817
(808) 586-5269 (V/TT)   FAX (808) 586-5377

Idaho
Commission for the Blind
341 West Washington
Boise, ID 83720-6000
(800) 542-8688   (208) 334-3220   FAX (208) 334-2963

Illinois
Bureau of Blind Services
Illinois Department of Rehabilitation Services
623 East Adams Street
PO Box 19429
Springfield, IL 62794-9429
(217) 782-2093   (217) 785-9328 (TT)   FAX (217) 524-1235

Indiana
Services for the Blind and Visually Impaired
402 West Washington Street, Room W453
PO Box 7083
Indianapolis, IN 46207-7083
(800) 545-7763   (317) 232-1433

Iowa
Department for the Blind
524 Fourth Street
Des Moines, IA 50309
(800) 362-2587   (515) 281-7999   (515) 281-1355 (TT)
FAX (515) 281-1263

Kansas
Division of Services for the Blind
Biddle Building, 2nd Floor
300 Southwest Oakley Street
Topeka, KS 66606-1995
(913) 296-4454 (V/TT)

Kentucky
Department for the Blind
427 Versailles Road
Frankfort, KY 40601
(800) 321-6668   (502) 564-4754   FAX (502) 564-3976

Louisiana
LA Rehabilitation Services
8225 Florida Boulevard, PO Box 94371
Baton Rouge, LA 70804-9371
(504) 925-4131   (504) 925-4178 (TT)

Maine
Bureau of Rehabilitation
Division for Blind and Visually Impaired
35 Anthony Avenue
Augusta, ME 04333-0011
(207) 624-5318

Maryland
Division of Rehabilitation Services
Maryland Rehabilitation Center
2301 Argonne Drive
Baltimore, MD 21218
(410) 554-3284   (410) 554-3277 (TT)   FAX (410) 554-3299

Massachusetts
Commission for the Blind
88 Kingston Street
Boston, MA 02111
(800) 392-6450   (800) 392-6556 (TT)   (617) 727-5550
FAX (617) 727-5960

Michigan
Commission for the Blind
201 North Washington, PO Box 30015
Lansing, MI 48909
(800) 292-4200   (517) 373-2062   (517) 373-4025 (TT)
FAX (517) 535-5829

Minnesota
Services for the Blind and Visually Handicapped
1745 University Avenue, West
St. Paul, MN 55104
(800) 652-9000   (612) 642-0500   (612) 642-0506 (TT)
FAX (612) 649-5927

Mississippi
Vocational Rehabilitation for the Blind
5455 Executive Place, PO Box 4872
Jackson, MS 39296-4872
(601) 364-2650   FAX (601) 364-2801

Missouri
Rehabilitation Services for the Blind
619 East Capitol Avenue
Jefferson City, MO 65101
(314) 751-4249   FAX (314) 751-4984

Montana
Visual Services Division
111 Sanders Street, PO Box 4210
Helena, MT 59604-4210
(406) 444-2590   FAX (406) 444-3632

Nebraska
Division of Rehabilitation Services for the Visually Impaired
4600 Valley Road
Lincoln, NE 68510-4844
(402) 471-2891 (V/TT)   FAX (402) 483-4184

Nevada
Bureau of Services to the Blind
Capitol Complex
505 East King, Room 503
Carson City, NV 89710
(702) 687-4444   (702) 687-4440 (TT)   FAX (702) 687-5980

New Hampshire
Bureau of Blind Services
78 Regional Drive, Building 2
Concord, NH 03301
(603) 271-3537   (603) 271-3471 (TT)   FAX (603) 271-1114

New Jersey
Commission for the Blind and Visually Impaired
153 Halsey Street, 6th Floor
PO Box 47107
Newark, NJ 07101
(800) 962-1233   (201) 648-3688   (201) 648-4559 (TT)
FAX (201) 648-7364

New Mexico
Commission for the Blind
PERA Building, Room 553
Santa Fe, NM 87503
(505) 827-4476   FAX (505) 827-4475

New York
Commission for the Blind and Visually Handicapped
Mailing address:
40 North Pearl Street
Albany, NY 12243-0001
Office:
Twin Towers, 1 Commerce Plaza
99 Washington Avenue, Room 724
Albany, NY 12210
(800) 342-3715   (518) 474-6812   FAX (518) 486-5819

North Carolina
Division of Services for the Blind
309 Ashe Avenue
Raleigh, NC 27606
(919) 733-9822   FAX (919) 733-9769

North Dakota
Office of Vocational Rehabilitation
400 East Broadway Avenue, Suite 303
Bismarck, ND 58501
(800) 472-2622   (701) 224-3999   (701) 224-3975 (TT)
FAX (701) 224-3976

Ohio
Bureau of Services for the Visually Impaired
400 East Campus View Boulevard
Columbus, OH 43235-4604
(800) 282-4536 (V/TT)   (614) 438-1255 (V/TT)   FAX (614) 438-1257

Oklahoma
Visual Services
300 Northeast 18th Street
Oklahoma City, OK 73105
(405) 424-3873   FAX (405) 521-4582

Oregon
Commission for the Blind
535 Southeast 12th Avenue
Portland, OR 97214
(503) 731-3218   (503) 731-3224 (TT)   FAX (503) 731-3230

Pennsylvania
Office for Blindness and Visual Services
1401 North Seventh Street, First Floor, PO Box 2675
Harrisburg, PA 17105
(800) 622-2842   (717) 787-6176   (717) 787-6280 (TT)

Puerto Rico
Vocational Rehabilitation Program
Box 1118
Hato Rey, PR 00919
(809) 725-1792   FAX (809) 721-6286

Rhode Island
State Services for the Blind and Visually Impaired
275 Westminster Street
Providence, RI 02903
(800) 752-8088   (401) 277-2382   (401) 277-3010 (TT)
FAX (401) 277-1328

South Carolina
Commission for the Blind
1430 Confederate Avenue
Columbia, SC 29201
(800) 922-2222   (803) 734-7520   FAX (803) 734-7885

South Dakota
Division of Service to Visually Impaired
East Highway 34, 500 East Capitol
Pierre, SD 57501-5070
(605) 773-4644   (605) 773-4544 (TT)   FAX (605) 773-5483

Tennessee
Services for the Blind
Citizens Plaza Building, 11th Floor
400 Deaderick Street
Nashville, TN 37219
(615) 741-2919   FAX (615) 741-4165

Texas
Commission for the Blind
4800 North Lamar
Austin, TX 78756
(800) 252-5204   (512) 459-2544   (512) 459-2573 (TT)
FAX (512) 459-2685

Utah
Division of Services for the Visually Handicapped
309 East 100th South
Salt Lake City, UT 84111
(800) 284-1823   (801) 533-9393 (V/TT)   FAX (801) 538-0437

Vermont
Division for the Blind and Visually Handicapped
Osgood Building
103 South Main Street
Waterbury, VT 05671-2301
(802) 241-2211   (802) 241-2400 (TT)   FAX (802) 244-8103

Virginia
Department for the Visually Handicapped
397 Azalea Avenue
Richmond, VA 23227
(800) 622-2155   (804) 371-3140 (V/TT)   FAX (804) 371-3351

Washington
Department of Services for the Blind
521 East Legion Way, PO Box 40933
Olympia, WA 98504-0933
(800) 552-7103   (206) 586-1224   (206) 586-6437 (TT)
FAX (206) 586-7627

West Virginia
Division of Rehabilitation Services
West Virginia Society for the Blind
State Capitol Complex
Charleston, WV 25305
(800) 642-3021   (304) 766-4600   (304) 766-4965 (TT)

Wisconsin
Office for the Blind
1 West Wilson Street
Madison, WI 53707
(608) 266-5600   (608) 266-9599 (TT)   FAX (608) 267-3657

Wyoming
Services for the Visually Handicapped
Room 144 Hathaway Building
Cheyenne, WY 82002
(307) 777-7274; 777-7256   FAX (307) 777-7234

APPENDIX B

DIVISION OFFICES OF
THE CANADIAN NATIONAL INSTITUTE FOR THE BLIND

<u>National Library</u>
1929 Bayview Avenue
Toronto, Ontario M4G 3E8
(416) 480-7520   FAX (416) 480-767

<u>Alberta - N.W.T.</u>
12010 Jasper Avenue
Edmonton, Alberta T5K 0P3
(403) 488-4871

<u>British Columbia - Yukon</u>
350 East 36th Avenue
Vancouver, British Columbia V5W 1C6
(604) 321-2311

<u>Manitoba</u>
1080 Portage Avenue
Winnipeg, Manitoba R3G 3M3
(204) 774-5421

<u>New Brunswick</u>
231 Saunders Street
Fredericton, New Brunswick E3B 1N6
(506) 458-0060

<u>Newfoundland and Labrador</u>
70 The Boulevarde
St. John's, Newfoundland A1A 1K2
(709) 754-1180

<u>Nova Scotia - Prince Edward Island</u>
6136 Almon Street
Halifax, Nova Scotia B3K 1T8
(902) 453-1480

Ontario
1929 Bayview Avenue
Toronto, Ontario M4G 3E8
(416) 486-2500

Quebec
1010, rue Ste-Catherine Est, Suite P-100
Montreal, Quebec H2L 2G3
(514) 284-2040

Saskatchewan
2550 Broad Street
Regina, Saskatchewan S4P 3Z4
(306) 525-2571

INDEX OF ORGANIZATIONS

This index contains organizations listed under sections titled "PROFESSIONAL ORGANIZATIONS," "RESEARCH ORGANIZATIONS," or "ORGANIZATIONS." These organizations may also be listed as vendors of publications, tapes, and other products.

Living with Low Vision: A Resource Guide for People with Sight Loss

A LARGE PRINT (18 point bold type) comprehensive directory that helps people with sight loss locate the services, products, and publications that they need to keep reading, working, and enjoying life. Chapters for children, elders, and people with both hearing and vision loss plus information on self-help groups, how to keep working with vision loss, and making everyday living easier. Third edition. $35.00

Providing Services for People with Vision Loss: A Multidisciplinary Perspective

Susan L. Greenblatt, Editor

Written by ophthalmologists, rehabilitation professionals, a physician who has experienced vision loss, and a sociologist, this book discusses how various professionals can work together to provide coordinated care for people with vision loss. Chapters include Vision Loss: A Patient's Perspective; Vision Loss: An Ophthalmologist's Perspective; Operating a Low Vision Aids Service; The Need for Coordinated Care; Making Referrals for Rehabilitation Services; Mental Health Services: The Missing Link; Self-Help Groups for People with Sight Loss; and Aids and Techniques that Help People with Vision Loss plus a Glossary. Also available on cassette. $19.95

Meeting the Needs of People with Vision Loss: A Multidisciplinary Perspective

Susan L. Greenblatt, Editor

Written by rehabilitation professionals, physicians, and a sociologist, this book discusses how to provide appropriate information and how to serve special populations. Chapters include What People with Vision Loss Need to Know; Information and Referral Services for People with Vision Loss; The Role of the Family in the Adjustment to Blindness or Visual Impairment; Diabetes and Vision Loss - Special Considerations; Special Needs of Children and Adolescents; Older Adults with Vision and Hearing Losses; Providing Services to Visually Impaired Elders in Long Term Care Facilities; plus a series of Multidisciplinary Case Studies. Also available on cassette. $24.95

Resources for Elders with Disabilities

This resource directory provides information about the services and products that elders with disabilities need to function independently. Printed in 18 point bold type, this book includes information on the diseases that cause common disabilities, the major rehabilitation networks, self-help groups, and laws that affect people with disabilities. Chapters on hearing loss, vision loss, diabetes, arthritis, osteoporosis, Parkinson's disease, falls, and stroke describe assistive devices, organizations, and publications that help people with these conditions. Second edition. $39.95

Meeting the Needs of Employees with Disabilities

A comprehensive resource guide that provides employers and counselors with the information they need to help people with disabilities retain or obtain employment. Includes information on government programs and laws such as the Americans with Disabilities Act, training programs, supported employment, transition from school to work, and environmental adaptations. Chapters on hearing and speech impairments, mobility impairments, visual impairment and blindness describe organizations, adaptive equipment, and services plus suggestions for a safe and friendly workplace. Individuals with disabilities also will find this to be a valuable resource guide. $42.95

Resources for People with Disabilities and Chronic Conditions

A comprehensive resource guide with chapters on spinal cord injury, low back pain, diabetes, multiple sclerosis, hearing and speech impairments, vision impairment and blindness, and epilepsy. Each chapter includes information about the disease or condition; psychological aspects of the condition; professional service providers; environmental adaptations; assistive devices; and descriptions of organizations, publications, and products. Chapters on rehabilitation services, independent living, and self-help, laws that affect people with disabilities (including the ADA), and making everyday living easier. Special information for children is also included. $44.95

LARGE PRINT PUBLICATIONS

Printed in 18 point bold type, these very special publications include information on each condition, rehabilitation services and professionals, products, and resources that help people with disabilities and chronic conditions to live independently. Titles include Living with Hearing Loss, Living with Arthritis, After a Stroke, Living with Diabetes, and Living with Low Vision. Printed on ivory paper with black ink for maximum contrast. 8 1/2" by 11" Sold in minimum quantities of 25 copies per title. See order form for complete list of titles and prices.

RESOURCES for REHABILITATION →

33 Bedford Street, Suite 19A • Lexington, MA 02173 • 617-862-6455 FAX 617-861-7517
Our Federal Employer Identification Number is 04-2975-007

NAME _____

ORGANIZATION _____

ADDRESS _____

PHONE _____

[ ] Check or signed institutional purchase order enclosed for full amount of order. Purchase orders accepted from government agencies, hospitals, and universities <u>only</u>.

[ ] Mastercard/VISA Card number: _____

Expiration date:_____ Signature: _____

ALL ORDERS OF $50.00 OR LESS <u>MUST</u> BE PREPAID.

TITLE	QUANTITY		PRICE	TOTAL
Living with low vision: A resource guide	____	X	$35.00	_____
Rehabilitation resource manual: VISION	____	X	39.95	_____
Providing services for people with vision loss	____	X	19.95	_____
Meeting the needs of people with vision loss	____	X	24.95	_____
Resources for people with disabilities and chronic conditions	____	X	44.95	_____
Meeting the needs of employees with disabilities	____	X	42.95	_____
Resources for elders with disabilities	____	X	39.95	_____

<u>MINIMUM PURCHASE OF 25 COPIES PER TITLE FOR THE FOLLOWING PUBLICATIONS</u>
Call for discount on purchases of 100 or more copies of any single title.

Living with low vision	____	X	2.00	_____
How to keep reading with vision loss	____	X	1.75	_____
Living with diabetic retinopathy	____	X	1.75	_____
Aging and vision loss	____	X	1.25	_____
Living with age-related macular degeneration	____	X	1.25	_____
Aids for everyday living with vision loss	____	X	1.25	_____
Living with arthritis	____	X	2.00	_____
Living with hearing loss	____	X	2.00	_____
After a stroke	____	X	2.00	_____
Living with diabetes	____	X	2.00	_____

SUB - TOTAL _____

SHIPPING & HANDLING: $25.00 or less, add $3.00; $25.01 to 50.00, add $5.00; $50.01 to 100.00, add $8.00; add $3.00 for each additional $100.00 or fraction of $100.00. For shipping to Alaska, Hawaii, U.S. territories, and Canada, add $3.00 to shipping and handling charges. Foreign orders must be prepaid in U.S. currency. Please write for shipping charges.   _____

TOTAL $_____

Prices are subject to change.